THE PROFESSIONAL DEVELOPMENT OF NURSING AND MIDWIFERY IN IRELAND

THE PROFESSIONAL DEVELOPMENT OF NURSING AND MIDWIFERY IN IRELAND

Key Challenges for the Twenty-First Century

YVONNE O'SHEA

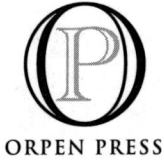

ORPEN PRESS

Published by
Orpen Press
Lonsdale House
Avoca Avenue
Blackrock
Co. Dublin
Ireland

e-mail: info@orpenpress.com
www.orpenpress.com

ISBN 978-1-871305-89-0

Printed in Ireland by SPRINT-print Ltd.

I would like to dedicate this book to two people. Firstly, to the memory of the late Mella Carroll (1934–2006), who, in addition to her distinguished career as a High Court judge in Ireland, was the chairperson of the Commission on Nursing. The Report of the Commission on Nursing *is without doubt the most influential and far-reaching publication in the history of the professions in Ireland. We all owe her a great debt of gratitude and may her memory live long.*

Secondly, I would also like to dedicate the book to Peta Taaffe, who, as Director of Nursing in St James's Hospital and as the first Chief Nursing Officer in Ireland, championed the development of the professions and pioneered many innovations that have in later years become part of the normal career pathway of nurses and midwives. She has been an inspiration to me and to many others.

TABLE OF CONTENTS

LIST OF TABLES

LIST OF FIGURES

LIST OF ABBREVIATIONS

ACS	acute coronary syndrome
AMAU	acute medical assessment units
AMNCH	Adelaide and Meath Hospital, Dublin, incorporating the National Children's Hospital
AMP	advanced midwife practitioner
AMR	antimicrobial resistance
AMU	acute medical units
ANP	advanced nurse practitioner
AP	advanced practitioner
BiPAP	bilevel positive airway pressure
BMI	body mass index
Board, the	Bord Altranais agus Cnáimhseachais na hÉireann, the Nursing and Midwifery Board of Ireland set up under the Nurses and Midwives Act 2011
CAIPE	Centre for the Advancement of Interprofessional Education
CAO	Central Applications Office
CEO	chief executive officer
CIM	clinicians in management
CME	centre for midwifery education
CMHT	community mental health team
CMM	clinical midwife manager
CMO	chief medical officer
CMS	clinical midwife specialist
CNE	centre for nurse education
CNM	clinical nurse manager
CNS	clinical nurse specialist
COPD	chronic obstructive pulmonary disease
CPAP	continuous positive airway pressure
CPD	continuing professional development
CS	clinical specialist

DALY	disability-adjusted life year
DCU	Dublin City University
DkIT	Dundalk Institute of Technology
DOMINO	domiciliary care in and out of hospital
DSIDC	Dementia Services Information and Development Centre
EC	European Commission
ECB	European Central Bank
ED	emergency department
EMP	emergency medicine programme
EQF	European Qualifications Framework
ESP	elective surgery programme
EU	European Union
EU-SILC	EU Survey on Income and Living Conditions
EWTD	European Working Time Directive
FIGO	International Federation of Gynaecologists and Obstetricians
FQEHEA	Framework of Qualifications of the European Higher Education Area
GDP	gross domestic product
GMS	general medical services
GNI	gross national income
GP	general practitioner
HCAI	healthcare-associated infection
HEA	Higher Educational Authority
HEI	higher education institute
HIQA	Health Information and Quality Authority
HIV/AIDS	human immunodeficiency virus infection/ acquired immunodeficiency syndrome
HPV	human papillomavirus
HRB	Health Research Board
HSE	Health Service Executive
HSRP	Health Service Reform Programme
ICM	International Confederation of Midwives
ID	intellectual disability
IDS-TILDA	Irish longitudinal study on ageing
IMB	Irish Medicines Board
IMF	International Monetary Fund
ISA	integrated service area
IT	information technology
IV	intravenous

IYJS	Irish Youth Justice Service
KPI	key performance indicator
LTSN	learning and teaching support network for health sciences and practice
MAU	medical assessment units
MDT	multidisciplinary team
MedEL	medicine for the elderly (clinical directorate)
MHC	Mental Health Commission
MidU	Midwifery-Led Unit Study
MLU	midwifery-led unit
MMR	measles, mumps and rubella (vaccine)
MWS	My World Survey
MWS-PSL	My World Survey – Post-Second-Level Education
MWS-SL	My World Survey – Second-Level Education
National Council	National Council for the Professional Development of Nursing and Midwifery
NCCP	national cancer control programme (HSE)
NCEC	National Clinical Effectiveness Committee
NCHD	non-consultant hospital doctor
NEHB	North Eastern Health Board
NFQ	National Framework of Qualifications
NHS	National Health Service (UK)
NIDD	national intellectual disability database
NIV	non-invasive ventilation
NMC	Nursing and Midwifery Council
NMPDU	Nursing and Midwifery Planning and Development Unit
NOCA	National Office of Clinical Audit
NPSDD	national physical and sensory disability database
NQAI	National Qualifications Authority of Ireland
NSRF	National Suicide Research Foundation
NTPF	National Treatment Purchase Fund
NUIG	National University of Ireland, Galway
OECD	Organisation for Economic Co-operation and Development
OHM	Office for Health Management
OMCYA	Office of the Minister for Children and Youth Affairs
OPAT	outpatient parenteral anti-microbial therapy

OPM	Office for Public Management
PAM	professionals allied to medicine
PCCC	primary, community and continuing care (of the HSE)
PCT	primary care trust (of the NHS)
PHN	public health nurse
QCCD	quality and clinical care directorate (of the HSE)
RCN	registered children's nurse
RCSI	Royal College of Surgeons in Ireland
RGN	registered general nurse
RM	registered midwife
RMHN	registered mental health nurse
RMI	Resource Management Initiative
RNID	registered nurse intellectual disability
RNP	registered nurse prescriber
RNT	registered nurse tutor
SDU	special delivery unit
SEA	Specify, Enable and Assure
SHA	Southern Health Area
SI	Statutory Instrument
TCD	Trinity College Dublin
TFR	total fertility rate
UCC	University College Cork
UCD	University College Dublin
UHI	universal health insurance
UK	United Kingdom
UL	University of Limerick
UN	United Nations
US	United States
WHO	World Health Organisation
WTE	whole time equivalents
X-ray	ionising radiation

ABOUT THE AUTHOR

Yvonne O'Shea, RGN, RM, RNT, BA (Health Management), MSc Econ (Public Policy), PhD, FFNM *ad eundem* (RCSI)

Yvonne O'Shea's career in nursing and midwifery has included experience in general nursing, midwifery, nurse education, nurse management, nurse regulation and professional development. Yvonne spent eleven years at St James's Hospital, Dublin, first as nurse tutor and subsequently as assistant director of nursing and nurse manager in the Crest Clinical Directorate. Yvonne was one of the first clinical directorate nurse managers in Ireland. During her time at St James's she was involved in a wide range of quality and standards development initiatives. She was nurse manager of the multidisciplinary team responsible for the successful bid to establish a new cardiac surgery unit in St James's Hospital and co-author of the successful tender document.

Since 1999, Yvonne has been at the forefront of leading nursing and midwifery in Ireland and implementing the vision for the professions contained in the *Report of the Commission on Nursing* (Government of Ireland, 1998). She was chief education officer at An Bord Altranais, where her achievements included the *Review of Scope of Practice for Nursing and Midwifery* and the introduction of the *Framework for the Scope of Nursing and Midwifery Practice*. Subsequently, as chief executive of the National Council for the Professional Development of Nursing and Midwifery, she was responsible for the development of a comprehensive clinical career pathway for nurses and midwives that has resulted in the creation of over 2,300 clinical nurse specialist/clinical midwife specialist posts, and 120 advanced nurse practitioner/advanced midwife practitioner posts. In addition, over 20,000 nurses and midwives have participated in additional professional development opportunities provided by the National Council. In cooperation with An Bord Altranais, she was instrumental in introducing the prescribing of medications by nurses and midwives (the Irish Medicines Board (Miscellaneous Provisions) Act 2006).

Yvonne is the author of *Nursing and Midwifery in Ireland: A Strategy for Professional Development in a Changing Health Service* (Blackhall Publishing, 2008) and *Clinical Directorates in the Irish Health Services: Managing Resources and Patient Safety* (Blackhall Publishing, 2009).

INTRODUCTION

This book sets out primarily to provide an overview of the many changes that have been taking place in the Irish health services and to show how these changes have affected and will continue to affect nurses and midwives and the professions of nursing and midwifery. It also sets out to show how nurses and midwives interact with others in the health services and how nursing and midwifery is a rich resource in the delivery of an efficient and effective healthcare service. The book continues a train of thought and reflection on nursing and midwifery that began with the publication of my first two books, *Nursing and Midwifery in Ireland: A Strategy for Professional Development in a Changing Health Service*[1] and *Clinical Directorates in the Irish Health Services: Managing Resources and Patient Safety*.[2] It also represents the culmination of my own personal and professional passion for nursing and midwifery that has driven me during more than 35 years of involvement in the professions in the areas of clinical nursing and midwifery, nurse education, professional regulation and, most recently, as chief executive of the National Council for the Professional Development of Nursing and Midwifery (the National Council).

This book is written for my colleagues who are working within the professions of nursing and midwifery in clinical, management, educational, research and policy-making settings. It is intended to provide them with an opportunity to appreciate the great strides that have been made in recent years, with the wish that what has been achieved is not lost in the maelstrom of change that lies ahead. It is also written for those thousands of young men and women who may be considering nursing and midwifery as a profession. It is my hope that they will be able to experience the extraordinary richness of the professions and perhaps be inspired to get involved. Ireland needs a cohort of professional, highly skilled and dedicated nurses and midwives to meet the challenges of the future.

The first two books were based on research I had carried out on professional development, resource management and clinical directorates. Among many other things, they included a description and analysis of the way in which the professions of nursing and midwifery had developed in Ireland as a result of the recommendations of the *Report of the Commission on Nursing* in 1998.[3] The books highlighted the changes that had taken place within the professions in response to the changing needs of society and the many changes that had occurred in the Irish health services as a result of a number of radical reform and transformation initiatives. They also described the major contribution that nursing and midwifery had already made to Irish health and the enhanced position they had achieved at the centre of the transformation of healthcare provision and patient safety.

Since 1998, as a result of the recommendations of the Commission on Nursing, there have been many changes within the professions of nursing and midwifery in Ireland. Among these changes, a comprehensive career pathway has been developed that has opened up many opportunities for nurses and midwives within the health services. Entry to the professions is now via a degree programme that has enjoyed major financial investment over the last fourteen years. The career path of nurses and midwives in Ireland today opens up rich opportunities for personal and professional development, from general practice to specialisation and advanced practice, and in areas such as clinical practice, research, education and management. Nurses and midwives are increasingly working in integrated care delivery settings and in many cases in a leading role in multidisciplinary teams.

In the short time since those books were published, Ireland as a country has undergone a radical transformation. We are living in a world that is only slowly recovering from the trauma of the worst global financial crash since the period of the Great Depression, which has shaken to its foundations our beliefs in our political systems, our financial and civic institutions and our cultural and social values. Over the last four years the Irish banking system collapsed and many people have seen their wealth disappear under the rubble of the burst property market bubble. The country is slowly emerging from a Programme of Recovery, referred to as 'the bailout', agreed with the International Monetary Fund, the European Central Bank and the European Commission. As a result, public expenditure is going through a reform programme, the like of which has never been witnessed in this country in the past. Every euro spent on services (including the health services) is examined for efficiency and effectiveness and value for money. Resources, and in particular human resources, are being depleted within the public services and public servants are being asked to do a lot more with fewer resources.

The Programme for Government (*Government for National Recovery 2011–2016*)[4] contains commitments that, if implemented, will result in significant changes in the way in which public services are delivered. In the health services, the Government is committed to a radical reform of institutions, practices and funding mechanisms.

In 2011, a new Nurses and Midwives Act[5] was enacted. The Act contained significant changes to the regulation of the professions of nursing and midwifery. The Act also dissolved the National Council, an agency that had been created on foot of a recommendation of the Commission on Nursing and that had been at the forefront of many of the professional developments that had taken place over the intervening fourteen years. In addition, the Department of Health is reviewing the undergraduate nursing and midwifery degree programme,[6] ten years after the introduction of the first degree programme and six years after the first cohort of graduates entered the workforce. It is clear that more changes lie ahead for the professions.

This book intends to address questions such as: How do we retain and build on what has been achieved over the last fourteen years since the publication of the *Report of the Commission on Nursing*? What provisions have been made to ensure that nursing and midwifery continue on a path of professional development in a manner that is best suited to the needs of the health services and its clients? How do we build on the best-practice standards that have been introduced in recent years in relation to the development and expansion of the roles of nursing and midwifery? What are the new challenges that face the professions within the health services of the future?

Chapter 1 of this book revisits an important theme for me. In my first book, published in 2008, I started off with an analysis of what I referred to as the *essence of nursing*. Four years later, despite the turbulence that surrounds us, I am more convinced than ever that there are core values and concepts that lie at the heart of the professions and that should remain constant. For that reason I have reproduced that chapter here at the beginning of this book.

The professions of nursing and midwifery face many challenges in the years ahead. There will be a need for strong leadership and a sure sense of the core values of the professions if a clear path is to be steered through what promise to be challenging times. The first chapter provides a reflection on the core values of the professions and sets the context for everything else that follows.

Chapter 2 provides a review of the state of the nation's health, looking at questions such as: How much do we spend on our health system? How many people are employed in the health services? What is happening to our population growth and to the levels of health in Ireland today? Against that backdrop, the evolution of our health services since the middle of the last century is described, with particular emphasis on the successive attempts at reform and transformation that have taken place over the last 25 years, culminating in a description of the most recent policy statements in relation to the future shape of the health services contained in the Programme for Government 2011[7] and the first signs of its implementation in 2012. The information contained in Chapter 2 is the essential social, economic and policy context within which the reflections on the professions of nursing and midwifery contained in the rest of the book need to be understood.

Chapter 3 looks at the statutory basis of the professions and how they are regulated. It also contains a description of the provisions of the Nurses and Midwives Act 2011 and the role of the regulatory body, the Nursing and Midwifery Board of Ireland. At the heart of the legislation is the pre-eminence of protection of the public, patient safety and quality in the regulation of the professions. This chapter also suggests how the development of specialisation and advanced practice within the professions should happen in the future in the wake of the dissolution of the National Council.

Chapter 4 describes and analyses the pre-registration and post-registration educational system which exists to underpin the professional status of nursing and midwifery. The chapter also includes reflections on how nurses and midwives need to maintain their professional competence over their lifetimes in light of the requirements of the Nurses and Midwives Act 2011. The chapter also examines the future of nursing and midwifery education, including a brief review of international trends in nursing and midwifery education.

Chapter 5 examines the career pathways that are open to nurses and midwives, how these pathways have been developed and how they should develop in the future. The development of roles, in particular where this requires expansion of practice, is examined in the light of the most recent guidance provided on this by the Department of Health.

Chapter 6 examines how the professions fit into the healthcare system as the most significant front-line resource in the provision of clinical care. It also examines the enormous challenges that lie ahead and the increasingly autonomous role that nurses and midwives are expected to fulfil as clinical leaders in the development, implementation and management of health services in Ireland.

Chapter 7 provides an analysis of three key concepts that are central to the integrity of all healthcare professions – accountability, clinical governance and leadership – and examines how these apply to nursing and midwifery. The professions of nursing and midwifery are evolving in Ireland through a period of constant change in the policy, fiscal and institutional environment. There is a much greater emphasis in this environment on transparency, openness and accountability.

Finally, Chapter 8 contains the results of a survey of nurses and midwives that I conducted in December 2011 as part of my research for this book. The survey covered the key concepts that are analysed throughout the book and examines the attitudes of senior nurse and midwife managers, educators and professional developers to the issues raised. The results provide much hope and encouragement for the future.

CHAPTER 1

The Core Values of Nursing and Midwifery

The foundations of modern professional nursing[8] can be traced back to 1860 and Florence Nightingale's classic *Notes on Nursing: What It Is and What It Is Not*.[9] In this publication, Nightingale spoke of nursing as aiding the reparative process of nature through the proper use of fresh air, light, warmth, cleanliness, quiet and the proper selection and administration of diet. She described nursing as the care that puts the patient in the best possible condition for nature to act. She also spoke of taking charge; that is, not just doing what is necessary oneself, but making sure that everyone else does so too. An essential feature of nursing is what she termed 'sound and ready observation'. This is a cumulative process that focuses on all parts of the body, cognisant of the fact that frequently patients cannot speak for themselves. Nightingale referred to this as 'the faculty of observation'. Sound and ready observation is, according to Nightingale, essential in a nurse. Thus it is through controlling the environment, providing a wide range of personal services, careful observation and taking charge that the nurse, according to Nightingale, aids the reparative process of nature.

Nightingale's view of nursing is still present in much of modern literature on the role of nurses and midwives, although the emphasis has shifted away from control of the environment to interaction with the individual. This may be because, in modern institutional settings, the nurse or midwife is less in control of the environment. In recent times, perhaps the most widely used definition of nursing is the one proposed by Virginia Henderson.[10] According to Henderson, the unique function of the nurse is to assist individuals, sick or well, in the performance of those activities contributing to health or its recovery (or to peaceful death) that they would perform unaided if they had the necessary strength, will or knowledge, and to do this in such a way as to help those who recover regain independence as soon as possible.

In 1995, a World Health Organisation (WHO) expert committee on nursing practice[11] considered Henderson's definition of nursing and concluded that, while the definition provided a sound foundation for describing nursing as it relates to individuals in a wide range of healthcare situations, it did not take account of issues arising from the changing orientations of health systems and policies or from the new roles and responsibilities that have evolved for nursing personnel. Nursing roles have changed in response to many factors, including technological advances, the transfer of tasks from medicine to nursing, the expansion of healthcare coverage through community nursing, the absence of physicians in some areas and the reorientation of healthcare systems to primary care. In response to these changes, the committee proposed the following three-part, functional description of nursing:

1. Nursing helps individuals, families and groups to determine and achieve their physical, mental and social potential, and to do so within the challenging context of the environment in which they live and work. The nurse requires competence to develop and perform functions that promote and maintain health as well as prevent ill health. Nursing also includes the planning and giving of care during illness and rehabilitation, and encompasses the physical, mental and social aspects of life as they affect health, illness, disability and dying.
2. Nursing promotes the active involvement of the individual and his or her family, friends, social group and community as appropriate, in all aspects of healthcare, thus encouraging self-reliance and self-determination while promoting a healthy environment.
3. Nursing is both an art and a science. It requires the understanding and application of specific knowledge and skills and it draws on knowledge and techniques derived from the humanities and the physical, social, medical and biological sciences.

The value of this contribution from WHO is that it provides a comprehensive description of the work of a nurse. It is a modern-day adaptation of the Nightingale view of the nurse and incorporates

Henderson's focus on the individual. It also emphasises the role of the nurse as an educator (of individuals and families) and a promoter of health, and the importance of knowledge and skills, science and expertise.

Other writers have provided deep insights into the philosophy and value system that underpins the role of the nurse. In 1999, Alison Kitson[12] identified what she described as the first essence or essential element in nursing: the philosophical and moral recognition of nursing as a person-centred activity. This is based on an acknowledgement of the uniqueness of the individual and the need for a set of attitudes and behaviours for the nurse to operate in a person-centred way. These include paying attention to detail; uncovering meaning in everyday situations; being attentive and available, reliable and true to promises; and understanding the importance of each person's own biography and how he or she is seeking to gain an understanding of what is happening to him or her.

Other commentators and theorists[13] have used a variety of approaches to explain how nurses can provide patient-centred care. These include the development of 'mutuality', or a demonstration of the nurse's ability to hold an unconditional positive regard for the other person.[14] It also includes being able to focus in on significant events, conditions or situations that enable the nurse to help each person feel intact.[15] Patricia Benner[16] elaborates on the powers of observation of the nurse and how these developed over time and experience to enable the 'expert' nurse to exercise 'clinical judgement' based on his or her experience and observations and to develop 'clinical wisdom'. It is part of the nurse's reflective practice. This, according to Kitson,[17] is part of a nurse's sensing and intuitive role, part of the shared experience between the nurse and the person who requires nursing, each one sharing the experience, each one recognising the contribution of the other. It is this philosophy, said Kitson, with which nursing should start and finish.

This complements, but perhaps goes further than, Nightingale's emphasis on 'sound and ready observation' as being essential in a nurse. Nightingale's emphasis was on observation of the physical environment and the physical well-being of the patient. In this case, it extends to the whole person and the human circumstances of the environment. It includes an element of relationship building as an essential requirement for the nurse to be able to contribute to an individual's ability to 'feel intact'.

In addition to this, however, Kitson said that nursing also requires a set of practical skills that constitute the essential elements that make up patient-centred care. These include:

1. **Essential care**: This includes putting the patient in the right environment to ensure optimal recovery. This is similar to Nightingale's emphasis on controlling the environment. It is perhaps the most important basic job of the nurse. It provides an answer to the key question, how can I ensure that the immediate environment is conducive to optimal care?
2. **Technological care**: This includes monitoring and observation skills, similar to Nightingale's 'sound and ready observation' and Benner's 'reflective practice' of the expert nurse as the basis for sound clinical judgement,[18] which requires an understanding of pathology, treatments, side-effects and potential hazards. This provides an answer to the question, how stable and predictable are the patient's physiological functions?
3. **Psychosocial/emotional care/information and education**: This includes interpersonal skills such as the ability to communicate, inform and educate patients, relatives and their carers. This provides an answer to the question, how stable and predictable are the patient's psychosocial and emotional states? It also provides an answer to the question, what does the patient need to know and learn about his or her condition or situation?
4. **Continuity and coordination**: This includes knowing how to provide a continuous, uninterrupted package of care, coordinated across geographic and service boundaries as well as between members of the healthcare team and the patient's own family (similar to what Nightingale referred to as 'taking charge'). This provides an answer to the question, how can I ensure that the patient experiences care that is uninterrupted and coordinated?

There are a number of common elements that run through these definitions and interpretations of nursing. Together, they make up what can be described as the essence of nursing, the core elements of which are:

1. **Person-centred care**: The individual experiences care in such a way as to feel that the nurse or midwife acts at all times in the interests of the person involved.

2. **Relationship-based care**: The experience of person-centred care is based on a relationship of empathy, of connection. The relationship is based on respect and consideration for the individual. It is animated by the values of equality, esteem, meaning, safety and trust.

3. **Holistic care**: The care provided by the nurse and midwife focuses on the totality of the person – physical, psychosocial and emotional. It is also sensitive to the cultural circumstances of the individual and is based on the value of respect for diversity.

4. **Education and promotion**: The care provided by the nurse or midwife is focused on promoting self-reliance and independence in individuals. This includes providing them with the wherewithal to be able to become independent. It extends beyond the individuals to their families and communities in order to ensure that support mechanisms are empowered to assist.

5. **Coordination**: Nurses and midwives ensure that individuals have access to whatever is required to assist them to achieve self-reliance and independence. This includes coordinating the inputs of other professionals, making technology available as required and taking charge of environmental management issues that affect the well-being of the individual.

6. **Knowledge-based care**: Nurses and midwives invest in their own education and development, fully aware that clinical wisdom comes about as a result of experience combined with knowledge and understanding. Competence development is an essential ingredient in the accountability values that nurses and midwives build into their professional practice. Nurses and midwives see themselves as professionals who combine science and art in the interests of individuals under their care.

A number of nursing theorists have sought to articulate this essence of nursing in the form of 'nursing models'. These models have served as a framework for developing the theory and practice of nursing.

The Neuman model of nursing[19] is a conceptual framework, or a visual representation, for thinking about patients and nurses and their interactions. This model views the person as a layered, multi-dimensional whole that is in constant dynamic interaction with the environment. The layers represent various levels of defence protecting the core being. The two major components in the model are stress reactions and systemic feedback loops. The patient/client reacts to stress with lines of defence and resistance. Continuous feedback loops fine-tune the lines of defence and resistance so as to achieve a maximal level of stability. The patient/client is in continuous and dynamic interaction with the environment. The exchanges between the environment and the patient/client are reciprocal, each one being influenced by the other. The goal is to achieve optimal system stability and balance. Prevention is the main nursing intervention to achieve this balance. Primary, secondary and tertiary prevention activities are used to attain, retain and maintain system balance.[20]

Patricia Benner takes the Dreyfus model of skill acquisition and applies it to nursing.[21] According to this model, nurses progress from being novices to experts principally though the knowledge they gain in the practice of nursing. In other words, the knowledge embodied in the practical world is important for the development of the nurse's skills and ability to care. His or her area of concern is not how to do nursing but, rather, 'how do nurses learn to do nursing?'

The Orem model of nursing was developed in 1985 by Dorothea Orem[22] and is also known as the 'self-care' model of nursing. It is used, in particular, in rehabilitation and primary-care settings where the patient is encouraged to be as independent as possible. The Orem model is based upon the philosophy that all 'patients wish to care for themselves'. Self-care requisites are groups of needs or requirements that Orem identified. They are classified as either universal self-care requisites (those needs that all people have), developmental self-care requisites (those needs that relate to development of the individual) or health deviation requisites (those needs that arise as a result of a patient's condition). When individuals are unable to meet their own self-care requisites, a self-care deficit occurs. It is the job of the nurse to determine these deficits and define a support modality based on an analysis of the dependency level of the individual. The support modality will be designed to provide either total compensation or partial compensation, or as an educative and supportive intervention.

The Roper–Logan–Tierney[23] model of nursing is a model of care based upon activities of living. The model is based loosely upon the activities of living evolved from the work of Virginia Henderson in 1966.[24] Roper and her colleagues listed twelve activities in which people engage in order to live. These are:

1. Maintaining a safe environment
2. Communication
3. Breathing

4. Eating and drinking
5. Elimination
6. Washing and dressing
7. Thermoregulation
8. Mobilisation
9. Working and playing
10. Expressing sexuality
11. Sleeping
12. Death and dying

These activities should be considered within the dependence–independence continuum. They are used to guide the initial assessment of a patient upon admission and are referred to again as the patient's condition is reviewed and the care plan revised. To provide effective care, all the patient's needs (which are identified by investigating the patient's specific requirements relative to each activity) must be met as practicably as possible. The model also incorporates a life-span continuum, where the individual passes from full dependence at birth, to full independence in midlife, returning to full dependence in old age or death.

Considered together, these models of nursing reveal the essence of nursing activity, namely, appropriate and responsive care of the patient's needs, and from that activity the identity of nursing may be deduced. They translate the essence of nursing into frameworks for theory and practice. They also serve to distinguish clearly the nursing model of care from the medical model.

The term 'medical model' was coined by the psychiatrist R.D. Laing[25] and denotes the set of processes and procedures in which all doctors are trained. This set includes complaint identification, history-taking, physical examination, ancillary tests if needed, diagnosis, treatment, and prognosis with or without treatment. The medical model aims to find medical treatments for diagnosed symptoms and syndromes and treats the human body as a very complex mechanism. It drives research and theorising about physical or psychological difficulties on the basis of causation and remediation. In this, it is quite distinct from the holistic approach of the nursing model, based on care for the needs of the individual and the development of a relationship within which this care is provided.

As nursing and midwifery move into areas of specialisation and advanced practice, it is important that the essence of nursing and midwifery is promoted and maintained. Thus, where the specialist or advanced practice is to be conducted in a particular area of clinical practice, what is required is a demonstration of the nursing and midwifery contribution to the area of practice.[26]

In developing areas of specialisation and advanced practice for nurses and midwives, therefore, it is important that the medical model does not dominate. It is equally important that an economic model of organisational and structural change within the health services does not dominate. Thus, for example, in developing the role of the nurse and midwife in the community, it is important that it is not driven solely by the need to achieve efficiencies or to substitute for the role of the general practitioner (GP) or other healthcare professionals. Nurses and midwives have an important part to play in adapting to the demands of efficiency and organisational change but must do so while remaining true to their own professional identity. It is only in this way that the professions of nursing and midwifery can make their own specific contribution to the health of individuals and their families in society.

At times of change it is important to have a touchstone that ensures that core values and ideals are not lost in the maelstrom of evolution and change. This is particularly important in nursing and midwifery in Ireland today, as it faces up to a future that holds many challenges, such as adaptation to new ways of working, new organisational structures, new relationships with other professionals and new social and cultural changes.

CHAPTER 2

The Irish Health Services

The State of the Nation's Health

In December 2011, the Department of Health published *Health in Ireland: Key Trends 2011*. This report presents a range of data on significant trends in health and healthcare over the past decade in Ireland[27] and covers population and health status as well as trends in service provision. The data paints a revealing picture of how far Irish health services have progressed over the last decade and how much of this progress is now being reflected in changing patterns of health and well-being, frequently for the better and sometimes for the worse.

Public Expenditure on Health

During the period generally regarded as the Celtic Tiger years (1995–2007), buoyant government revenues, especially substantial taxes from a booming construction sector, enabled the Government to significantly increase public health spending, from around €3 billion in 1995 to over €14 billion in 2007. With the collapse of the construction boom, the Irish economy went into recession in 2008. There was a time lag before the resulting government spending cuts took effect, so Irish healthcare spending actually increased in 2008 and 2009, when it peaked at €15.4 billion. In 2010, health spending fell to €14.8 billion and fell further to an estimated €14 billion in 2011. While public health expenditure has been cut in line with the new economic and fiscal realities, the demand for health services has increased, fuelled by, among other things, a continuing growth in population, a high fertility rate, and people living longer and the consequential increase in the number of older people in the general population.

The legacy of the boom years, as far as the health services is concerned, is a greatly increased level of investment in the health services. Over the last three years, however, it has become evident that much of this is not sustainable, particularly in the area of capital expenditure. Public capital expenditure on health was €366 million in 2010, representing an 18 per cent decline on the previous year and an overall decrease to 2001 levels.

Total public non-capital expenditure on health has increased by 72.7 per cent since 2002; however, it has decreased by 5.2 per cent between 2010 and 2011. In 2009, Ireland's total expenditure on health was 9.5 per cent of gross domestic product (GDP) and 11.4 per cent of gross national income (GNI). This compares with the Organisation for Economic Co-operation and Development (OECD) averages of 9.6 per cent and 10.2 per cent respectively. Ireland's per capita total health expenditure increased steadily in real terms between 2001 and 2008, and decreased between 2008 and 2009.

Employment in the Health Services

One of the more revealing sets of statistics that illustrate the level of increased investment in Irish health services over the past decade is the number of people employed in the services. Between 2000 and 2009, employment in the public health services increased by nearly 39 per cent of whole time equivalents (WTE). All categories of staff experienced increases, but the largest rise, of 110 per cent, to about 16,000 WTE, was in the category of health and social care professionals. These included clinical biochemists, physiotherapists, dieticians, psychologists, medical scientists, radiographers, occupational therapists, social care workers, orthoptists, social workers, podiatrists, and speech and language therapists.

Since 2007, in the wake of the collapse of the Celtic Tiger economy in Ireland, total numbers employed in the public health services have shown a gradual decline. Between 2010 and 2011, the largest fall in numbers has been in the management/administration category, reducing by 7.2 per cent.

The number of medical consultants employed by the public health service increased by almost 45 per cent in the period 2002–2011. They also increased by almost 3 per cent between December 2010 and September 2011. Medical and dental were the only grade category to show an increase between December 2010 and September 2011. The number of non-consultant hospital doctors (NCHDs) increased by almost 16 per cent in the period 2002–2011. They also increased slightly between December 2010 and September 2011. The numbers of general medical service general practitioners (GMS GPs) (i.e. participants in the Choice of Doctor Scheme) has increased by 44 per cent since 1998.

Employment of nurses and midwives increased by 7.8 per cent between 2002 and 2011, from 33,395 to 35,993. Nurses and midwives make up the largest grade category in the public health service, accounting for 35 per cent of total staff employed. Employment of nurses and midwives within the services reached its peak in 2007 at 39,006. Since then, numbers have declined by 7.7 per cent, reverting employment levels in nursing and midwifery to approximately where they were in 2005. These reductions are indicative of the decisions that have been taken to curb the overall level of public expenditure within the health services in recent years.

A lot of care is provided in Ireland by unpaid carers. The Central Stastics Office (CSO)[28] estimates that there are over 187,000 carers providing unpaid care in our communities. *The National Carers' Strategy – Recognised, Supported, Empowered,*[29] published by the Department of Health in 2012, recognises this fact. We will return to further consideration of this important part of our healthcare system in Chapter 6.

The increases in the numbers of social care professionals, consultants and NCHDs are a reflection of the impact of the various strategies that were introduced over the period aimed at reforming the health services. A central part of this reform was the introduction of consultant-led services, supported by appropriately qualified clinical personnel in a wide range of disciplines. This period saw the emergence of multidisciplinary integrated teams working across institutional boundaries and, increasingly, in specialised directorates with a clinical professional at the top. These developments will be described in the next section of this chapter, which deals with the evolution of the Irish health services.

Changing Demographics

The changes in the health services were also driven by rapidly changing demographics in Ireland. Census 2011 results[30] show that Ireland's population has continued to grow strongly since Census

2006, increasing by 348,404 to 4,588,252. This is an increase of 8.2 per cent over the 2006 Census, an annual average increase of 1.6 per cent. The previous annual average increase between Census 2002 and Census 2006 was 2.1 per cent, the highest on record. Looking back over twenty years, Ireland's population has increased by over one million, or 30.1 per cent. Over the past 60 years, the population has increased by 1.6 million, or 55 per cent. Growth of these proportions in the population gives some indication of the dynamic nature of Irish society during those years of unprecedented change.

Despite the traumatic changes brought about by the economic collapse of recent years, Ireland continued to enjoy a very strong growth in its population, as evidenced by the numbers of births in each year. During 2010, there were 73,724 births recorded in Ireland. This represents a 1 per cent decrease on the previous year, but there are still around 15,000 more births per year than a decade ago. The total fertility rate[31] (TFR) has remained steady at 2.07. However, Ireland continues to have the highest rate of fertility amongst European Union (EU) countries, the EU average being 1.57.

Ireland is now beginning to catch up with other European countries in terms of population ageing. The number of people in older age groups is beginning to increase significantly. The number of people over the age of 65 years will more than double within the next 30 years to over one million, with the largest proportional increase in the 85+ age category.

Life Expectancy

Over the past decade, Ireland has achieved a rapid and unprecedented improvement in life expectancy. During a period when the average life expectancy in the EU has continued to rise, life expectancy in Ireland has increased from nearly one year below the EU average life expectancy to just above it. Much of this increase is due to significant reductions in major causes of death, such as circulatory system diseases. When life expectancy is expressed as years lived in good health (i.e. healthy life years), the difference between women and men is much less significant, indicating that women live longer but with more health problems.

In addition to living longer, Irish people also have a very high perception of the quality of their own health. Ireland continues to have the highest levels of self-perceived good health of those countries in Europe participating in the EU Survey on Income and Living

Conditions (EU-SILC). In 2009, 84 per cent of males and 83 per cent of females rated their health as being good or very good. This is the highest in the EU and compares with an average of 71 per cent and 65 per cent for males and females respectively across the EU. Self-perceived good health is related to income levels, with 20 per cent more people in the highest income group rating their health good or very good compared with the lowest income group.

Chronic Diseases

However, the survey shows significant chronic health problems in the older age groups, with around half of those aged 65+ reporting a chronic illness or condition. Twenty-nine per cent of people who report having a disability stated they have felt worn out all or most of the time, compared with 11 per cent of those without a disability. Almost 47 per cent of males and 54 per cent of females aged 65 and over reported suffering from a chronic illness or condition. In the 75+ age category, 44 per cent and 59 per cent of males and females respectively reported some limitation in activity due to health problems. Seven per cent of adults reported having ever been diagnosed with asthma. A detailed international review of the prevalence of chronic diseases was conducted by the World Health Organisation (WHO) in 2010.[32] We will return to a more detailed analysis of this in Chapter 6, when we examine the challenges facing nurses and midwives in the health services today.

Death Rates

As we are living longer, it is no surprise to find that death rates in Ireland have also declined. Over the ten-year period 2001–2010, age-standardised mortality rates[33] for all causes fell by 28 per cent. Most recently, death rates declined by almost 9 per cent between 2009 and 2010. Diseases of the circulatory system accounted for almost 34 per cent of all deaths registered in 2010. A decline in the age-standardised death rate of over 39 per cent occurred between 2001 and 2010. There has been a 15 per cent decline in the age-standardised death rate for malignant neoplasms during the period 2001–2010. The female breast cancer death rate declined by 24 per cent during the same period.

Death rates from suicide are down 19 per cent since 2001 and decreased by 6 per cent between 2009 and 2010. In 2011, however, the number of suicides rose by 7 per cent,[34] as a total of 439 men and 86 women were recorded as having taken their own lives, the majority of whom were aged between 15 and 44. The increase, according to commentators, was directly attributable to the impact the recession was having on mental health, especially of young men.[35]

Ireland's age-standardised death rate in 2009 was 1.5 per cent below the EU average. For the same period the death rate from all cancers was 7.7 per cent above the EU average. Five-year relative survival rates from selected cancers remain lower in Ireland than the average for OECD countries. However, the gap is significantly narrowing, particularly for breast and cervical cancers.

Lifestyle

Figure 1 contains data published by the Department of Health and Children[36] showing trends for both alcohol and cigarette consumption over the period 1991–2010. Over the whole period, alcohol consumption increased from 10 to 12 litres per person aged over 15 years of age. It declined from a high of 14 litres per person aged over 15 years during the decade 2002 to 2012. Over the same period, consumption of cigarettes declined from approximately 2,300 cigarettes per year per person aged over 15 years to about 1,200. The sharpest decline has occurred since 2003, when consumption was still in excess of 2,000 cigarettes per year per person aged over 15 years. However, the official figures for alcohol consumption do not include purchases made outside the State or illegal imports into the State, which may exaggerate the decline. According to a report published in 2012 by the Alcohol Beverage Federation of Ireland,[37] the average alcohol consumption per person fell in the last decade to 12 litres per person per year, 17 per cent below the 2001 peak. However, the report states that caution should be exercised in reading the decline as a positive indicator of alcohol consumption in Ireland, as an increase in excise duty in 2003, allied to the fact that one person in five does not drink alcohol, could have an important influence on these figures.

According to the report, average alcohol consumption declined from its peak in 2001 of 14.4 litres per adult per year to 13.5 litres per adult per year in 2003. It broadly stayed at this level until 2007, and in 2008 it declined to 12.5 litres per adult per year. There was a further decline in 2009, followed by an increase in 2010 and no change in 2011 (at 12 litres). The report points out that the 2009 and

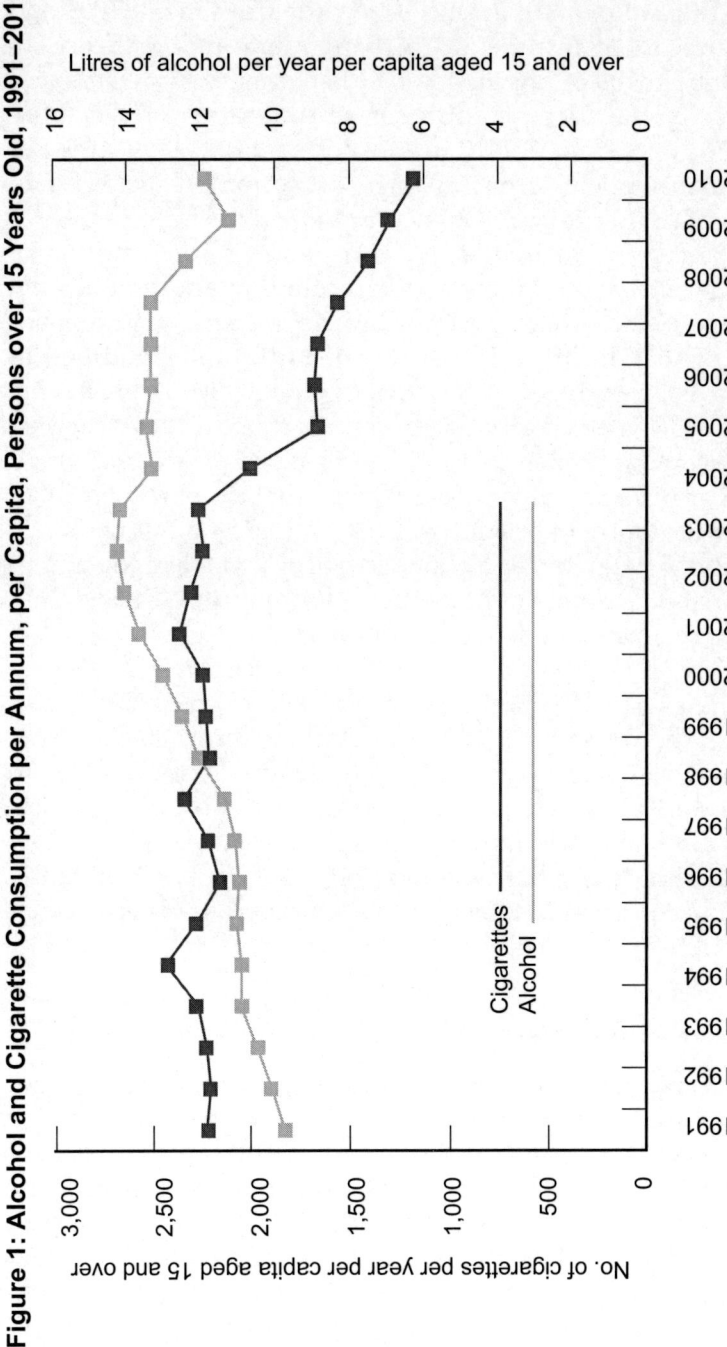

Figure 1: Alcohol and Cigarette Consumption per Annum, per Capita, Persons over 15 Years Old, 1991–2010

Litres of alcohol per year per capita aged 15 and over

No. of cigarettes per year per capita aged 15 and over

Cigarettes
Alcohol

Source: Revenue Commissioners Statistical Reports; CSO (population data)
Note: Alcohol is measured in terms of pure alcohol consumed, based on sales of beer, cider, wine and spirits

2010 figures were influenced by the changing level of cross-border purchases of alcohol and part of the recorded decline in 2009 and part of the recorded increase in 2010 are due to this influence. In addition, the census of population had been revised upwards and this will lower the average adult consumption for each of those years, with the revised 2011 figure expected to be 11.8 litres per adult. In international terms, average consumption increased in several OECD countries but declined in Ireland over the period.[38]

Public perception in Ireland of Irish people's consumption of alcohol, however, would appear to indicate that abuse of alcohol is a serious social problem. According to a survey carried out on behalf of the Health Research Board (HRB) and published in a report in 2012 entitled *Alcohol: Public Knowledge, Attitudes and Behaviours*,[39] the vast majority (86 per cent) of those surveyed agreed that there were high rates of drunkenness on Irish streets at night and a similar majority (85 per cent) agreed that the current level of alcohol consumption in Ireland was too high. Seven out of ten (71 per cent) did not agree that alcohol consumption was reducing in Ireland. A similar number (73 per cent) thought that Irish society tolerated high levels of alcohol consumption.

In August 2012, the Global Adult Tobacco Survey (GATS) Collaborative Group[40] published in *The Lancet* the results of a survey of tobacco use by 3 billion individuals from 16 countries. The survey was based on an analysis of nationally representative cross-sectional household surveys. The surveys showed high rates of smoking in men, early initiation of smoking in women and low quit ratios, reinforcing the view that efforts to prevent initiation and promote cessation of tobacco use are needed to reduce associated morbidity and mortality.

Activity Levels in the Health Services

One of the important developments in Irish health services over the past decade has been the move to reduce the length of stay by patients in acute hospitals and shift towards day-care services, not involving a hospital stay, increased outpatient services and the provision of more care in the community. This trend can be seen in the statistics. Total hospital discharges continue to rise, but an increasing proportion of this activity (60 per cent in 2010) is now carried out on a day-care basis. The average length of stay in hospital for inpatients has fallen to 5.9 days for the first time. Inpatient discharges from publicly funded acute hospitals have increased by almost 10 per cent since 2001 but remained static between 2009 and 2010. Day cases have increased by 119 per cent since 2001 and have also increased by 4.7 per cent between 2009 and 2010. Improved and less invasive medical practice is largely responsible for the rapid growth in day patient activity.

Since 2008, the number of day cases (excluding dialysis) treated in publicly funded acute hospitals has been higher than the number of inpatients. This gap has increased every year since 2008. Emergency department (ED) attendances decreased by nearly 2 per cent between 2009 and 2010. Over the same period, outpatient attendances increased by 5 per cent. Long-stay care in hospitals and other healthcare institutions is increasingly dominated by older age groups. Those aged 85 and over in long-stay care as a percentage of all those in long-stay care has increased by 21 per cent during the period 2001–2010. All other age groups over 65 have shown declines over the same period.

In the area of psychiatric services, successive governments since 1984 have emphasised the importance of shifting services away from long-stay institutional settings into the community. The impact of this approach is evident in the statistics. The number of admissions to psychiatric hospitals and units has continued to decline, with a decrease of 3 per cent between 2009 and 2010. There are now almost 20 per cent fewer admissions than in 2001. The number of persons with an intellectual disability (ID) availing of day services has increased by 15 per cent for day attendees and decreased almost 2 per cent for full-time residents over the period 2001–2010.

Children

Some worrying trends emerged during the last decade in relation to the health of children. The Growing Up in Ireland[41] study reported that 26 per cent of nine-year-old children were found to have a body mass index (BMI) that was outside of the 'healthy' range. Of these, 19 per cent were defined as overweight and 7 per cent as obese. In addition, the number of children in care increased by 28 per cent between 2000 and 2009. The percentage of these children in foster care also increased over the same period by 16 per cent. Nearly 90 per cent of children in care are now being fostered. On a more positive note, immunisation rates have been increasing since 2002 and are now approaching the 95 per cent rate envisaged by the *Immunisation Guidelines for Ireland*.[42] The immunisation uptake rates of children aged 24 months in 2010 was 94 per cent for most immunisations, with the exception of the MMR, Meningococcal and Pneumococcal Conjugate. Hepatitis B and Pneumococcal Conjugate vaccines were introduced in 2008 and show immunisation rates of 94 per cent and 88 per cent respectively.

General Medical Services

Finally, the level of activity in the GMS is an indicator of the health status of those in possession of medical cards in Ireland. In 2010, 86 per cent of those with a medical card reported visiting a GP at least once in the previous twelve months, compared with 73 per cent for those with private health insurance and 57 per cent for those with neither. The average number of GP consultations was also higher among medical cardholders in all age groups. Between 2009 and 2010 there was a 9 per cent increase in medical cards to over 1.6 million, representing 36 per cent of the population. The number of GP-visit cards increased by 19 per cent to nearly 118,000. The number of prescription items dispensed under the GMS increased by over 5 per cent between 2008 and 2009, while the average cost per item also increased. The costs of the GMS and the phenomenon of a two-tiered system of health with many built-in inequalities are themes that will re-emerge as we analyse throughout this book emerging policies and the challenges that have presented themselves in recent years.

The Evolution of the Irish Health Services

Health policy was not a priority for Irish governments until the late 1940s. It was not until 1947 that the Irish Government established a separate Department of Health. Until then, health had been a matter for local government to organise. With the Health Act 1970,[43] control of the health services was removed from the local authority system and reorganised as eight regional health boards under the ultimate control of the Department of Health. However, the modern reform of the Irish health services can be said to have begun with the publication by the Department of Health in 1994 of an ambitious strategy, *Shaping a Healthier Future: A Strategy for Effective Healthcare in the 1990s*.[44] The strategy was based on three basic principles:

equity, quality and accountability. The strategy was founded on the thinking contained in a number of earlier health policy documents. These included *Health: The Wider Dimensions* (1986),[45] a response to the World Health Organisation's programme, *Global Strategy for Health for All by the Year 2000* (1981);[46] the *Report of the Commission on Health Funding* (1989);[47] the Kennedy *Reports of the Dublin Hospitals Initiative Group* (1991);[48] the Hickey report on *Community Medicine and Public Health* (1990);[49] and others.

In 2001, the Department of Health and Children published a new strategy, *Quality and Fairness: A Health System for You*,[50] which outlined a ten-year programme of investment and reform of the health system. It was built on the planned and strategic approach of the previous health strategy, as well as a number of other health-related strategies. The earlier strategy, *Shaping a Healthier Future*, was based on the three principles of equity, quality and accountability. *Quality and Fairness* added a fourth – people-centredness. The strategy was further developed through a number of significant studies aimed at introducing the necessary reforms in key areas of the services:

- The *Report of the National Task Force on Medical Staffing* (the Hanly Report)[51] addressed the issues facing the acute hospital system.
- The *Report of the Commission on Financial Management and Control Systems in the Health Service* (the Brennan Report)[52] addressed the way in which the services are funded.
- *Primary Care: A New Direction*,[53] produced by the Department of Health and Children, addressed the issues facing primary care.
- *Action Plan for People Management*,[54] produced by the Department of Health and Children and the Health Service National Partnership, responded to the key questions of human resource management.
- *Health Information: A National Strategy*,[55] produced by the Department of Health and Children, examined issues of information and quality within the services.
- The *Audit of Structures and Functions in the Health System 2003*,[56] prepared by Prospectus Strategy Consultants (the Prospectus Report), tackled the difficult and complex area of organisational reform and proposed the establishment of the Health Service Executive (HSE), replacing the old health boards that had been established in 1970.

Based on the findings of the recommendations that emerged from these studies, the Government introduced the Health Service Reform Programme (HSRP),[57] in 2003. At the time, it was seen as the most ambitious programme of change for the Irish health system in over 30 years. The programme was backed by a significant level of State investment: as noted earlier, health expenditure in Ireland had increased from €3.7 billion in 1997 to €15.4 billion in 2009.[58]

The Health Act 2004[59] established the Health Service Executive (HSE), which came into operation in January 2005, with responsibility for the management and delivery of health and personal social services in the Republic of Ireland. According to the Act, the objective of the HSE is 'to use the resources available to it in the most beneficial, effective and efficient manner to improve, promote and protect the health and welfare of the public'.[60] The HSE was given responsibility for integrating the delivery of health and personal social services and it replaced the previous structure of regional health boards, the Eastern Regional Health Authority and a number of other agencies and organisations. The HSE was then (and still is) the largest organisation in the State, employing over 130,000 people.[61]

The basis of the HSRP is the separation of policy formulation from service delivery. The creation of the HSE involved a complete separation of policy and executive functions: responsibility for policy formulation and monitoring was the role of the Department of Health and Children; responsibility for the executive day-to-day management of the health services was the role of the HSE. The Department of Health and Children was responsible for monitoring and evaluating the work of the HSE and its expenditure. The HSE would, in turn, manage the health service as a single national entity and would also provide advice to the Minister and contribute to policy formulation. This approach was in line with the broad policy principle that Government Ministers should divest themselves of executive functions and focus on policy and planning.

The health strategy, *Quality and Fairness*, highlighted the key role of clinicians (doctors, nurses, and health and social care professionals) in the planning and delivery of a quality, patient-centred health service, particularly in relation to transparency and accountability. A central component of the role is to create and maintain effective working partnerships between clinicians and managers. This was the basis of the clinicians in management (CIM) initiative, which was launched by the Department of Health and Children in 1998 to

strengthen the involvement of key health professionals in the planning and management of services.[62] CIM was initially introduced
in five pilot sites in Irish hospitals, and in 1999 there was a second-
wave rollout of CIM into seventeen additional hospitals, which was
then further increased to thirty-one.

The CIM initiative heralded the biggest change to the management of Irish hospitals for many years. It was designed with one
primary objective: to improve the quality of care available to hospital patients. The aim of the initiative was to provide for balanced
involvement in decision making between doctors, nurses and allied
health professionals, and to decentralise the responsibility for
managing resources down to local units with their direct participation. It sought to build a sense of equal partnership between the
various professional groups within the hospital and give them a
common focus on improving patient care.

In its 2006 National Service Plan,[63] the HSE said that it would
develop models of team-working, including further development
of CIM, to contribute to enhanced team-working and service delivery, with models for each service developed and implementation
plans agreed. CIM became closely aligned with the concept of
clinical directorates[64] and the clinical directorate concept became
the explicit HSE instrument for directly involving clinicians in the
management of a hospital or operational area.

In December 2006, the HSE launched its *Transformation
Programme 2007–2010,*[65] and its *Corporate Plan 2008–2011*[66] proposed
to engage with staff and create work environments that support
transformation. The Corporate Plan said that services would
move to a consultant-delivered rather than a consultant-led acute
service, functioning within a well-developed clinical directorate
structure. There would be more clinical involvement in the design
and management of health and personal social services, with a
move to a consultant-delivered rather than a consultant-led acute
service, functioning within a well-developed clinical directorate
structure.

Clinical directorates represent an approach to the management of
health services that is now quite common in the healthcare systems
of many developed economies. It is based on the involvement of
clinicians in making decisions about the choices involved in how
resources should be used.[67] Decisions about how best to use these
resources can make the difference between life and death for individual clients of the health services. The use of clinical directorates

as a model of management and decision making is based on the premise that those who make decisions about the use of the resources that are available should include those who possess the knowledge about how resources can be used to best effect. Clinical leadership and team-based service delivery would be embedded in the organisation.

The Transformation Programme recognised that the development of clinical directorates would represent a major step forward in the management and development of public healthcare in Ireland. In order to introduce clinical directorates and related systems of clinical leadership, achieving agreement on a new contractual framework for consultants was a key objective of the HSE. The HSE agreed a new contract with the Irish Medical Organisation and the Irish Hospital Consultants' Association in 2008 that included provision for the introduction of clinical directorates. The contract recognised the importance of the role of clinical director, which placed consultants within the leadership structure in the management of the health services. The contract came into effect in January 2009.[68] The first 40 appointments of clinical directors were made in January 2009.[69]

In July 2008 the HSE published an integrated services programme[70] that involved major organisational changes. The reorganisation was aimed at providing more local responsibility and authority within defined national parameters, more robust area structures and more clinical involvement in the design and management of health and social services, as well as accelerating the integration of primary, community and acute care. A new regional structure would have all services administered locally in specified geographical areas. Within the HSE, a new national director of quality and clinical care would drive clinical governance, quality and risk, define national clinical standards and protocols, and ensure engagement with clinical stakeholders. A single national directorate of integrated service delivery would have operational responsibility for all hospital- and community-based services. A national director of planning would lead integrated service planning. As part of the Integrated Services Programme, and within the terms of the new contract, the HSE announced plans for the introduction of clinical directors throughout the health services on a two-year phased basis.[71] Among other objectives, the new structure was intended to provide clinical engagement at all levels and the facility for front-line clinicians and other professionals to make effective local decisions.

Building a Culture of Patient Safety, the report of the Commission on Patient Safety and Quality Assurance,[72] chaired by Dr Deirdre Madden, was published in 2008 in response to the findings of the Lourdes Hospital Inquiry[73] and to health system failures in other jurisdictions. The Commission was established in 2007, comprising representatives from medicine, nursing, management and patient groups, and was charged with developing proposals on patient safety and quality in healthcare. The Commission's report referred to incidents in Ireland relating to the misdiagnosis of cancer that point strongly to poor management, governance and communications, especially in circumstances where a serious adverse event takes place.[74] Patient safety had become a national and international imperative in the years leading up to the report, with increased emphasis around the world on patient safety in policy reform, legislative changes and development of standards of care driven by quality-improvement initiatives. The report pointed out that, despite a professionally trained and highly motivated workforce in the health system and huge investment in healthcare services in recent years, the Irish healthcare system lacked a framework aimed at reducing the likelihood of errors occurring and responding to errors. The report also stated that there had not been sufficient regulation in place to ensure as far as possible that patients receive the highest possible quality of care.

The report said that good governance structures in healthcare should focus on patient safety and noted that one structural suggestion to develop this focus was to organise clinicians into groups of patient-focused service configurations, commonly known as clinical streams or clinical directorates. The HSE had at this time already begun the systematic introduction of clinical directorate structures throughout the health services.

In response to recommendations in the report, in September 2010 the Patient Safety First Initiative[75] was launched. A key component of this initiative was the National Framework for Clinical Effectiveness, the purpose of which was to provide formal structures and processes to support clinical effectiveness. Clinical effectiveness involves a number of processes but primary among these are the development or adaptation and use of clinical guidelines to support evidence-based practice and the use of clinical audits to improve patient care and outcomes. The oversight of the National Framework for Clinical Effectiveness was provided by the National Clinical Effectiveness Committee (NCEC). The NCEC provides guidance to clinical guideline development groups on how to develop clinical guidelines. In 2011, the NCEC published Interim Guidance for Clinical Guideline Development Groups.[76]

In 2007 the Health Information and Quality Authority (HIQA) was established with the purpose of driving improvements in Ireland's health and social care services. It is responsible for quality and safety in Ireland's health and social care services through setting standards in health and social services; monitoring health-care quality; providing a health and social services inspectorate; monitoring and encouraging developments in health technology; and improving the quality of health information.

Reporting to the Minister for Health, the role of HIQA is to 'promote safety and quality in the provision of health and personal social services for the benefit of the health and welfare of the public'.[77] It sets national standards for the provision of health and social care services (except for mental health services, which are the responsibility of the Mental Health Commission) in Ireland. These incorporate minimum standards for quality and safety for a given service, and developmental standards to support moving towards excellence, based on evidence and best practice within Ireland and internationally. HIQA continuously monitors services to ensure that the standards are being met. Standards are monitored by multidisciplinary teams of professional and lay reviewers undertaking site visits and working with healthcare organisations to identify areas for improvement. The teams also recognise good practice. Quality assurance review reports are published on the HIQA website, together with an action plan from the service provider outlining a programme to address the recommendations of the report.

As part of HIQA's commitment to the Patient Safety First Initiative, in 2010 it published its *Draft National Standards for Safer and Better Healthcare: Consultation Document*.[78] In publishing the document, HIQA pointed out that it had the remit for setting standards for quality and safety in healthcare services under section 8 of the Health Act 2007.[79] This includes services provided or funded by the HSE. The consultation document presented for public consultation a set of proposed new national standards for the quality and safety of healthcare services in Ireland.

In June 2012 HIQA published the final approved version of the national standards. Two publications were presented: *A Guide to the National Standards for Safer Better Healthcare*[80] and *National*

Standards for Safer Better Healthcare.[81] The national standards had been designed to describe the principles of how healthcare should be provided in any care setting. HIQA indicated that it would monitor compliance with these national standards and they would form the basis for future licensing of healthcare facilities. Service users, including patients, carers, families and representatives, could use the national standards to help them understand what high-quality and safe healthcare should be and what they should expect from a well-run service. It was intended that this information would help service users to voice their expectations of healthcare services. The national standards were also to provide a sound basis for anyone planning, funding or providing healthcare services to work towards achieving and maintaining high-quality, safe and reliable care.

In May 2012 HIQA published what is likely to become a landmark report on the quality, safety and governance of healthcare in Ireland. The report was the outcome of an investigation into the care provided for patients who require acute admission by the Adelaide and Meath Hospital incorporating the National Children's Hospital (AMNCH).[82] The AMNCH is commonly known as Tallaght Hospital, and the report is referred to as the Tallaght Hospital Report.[83] A more detailed analysis of the content and implications of this report is provided in Chapter 7 of this book.

The full implementation of a robust quality, safety and risk management programme is one of the strategic objectives identified in the HSE's *Corporate Plan 2008–2011*.[84] The plan proposed to establish a quality and clinical care directorate (QCCD) headed by a national director of quality and clinical care. This was intended to develop clinical leadership and clinical governance across the HSE and facilitate consolidation of the work carried out to date on the quality, safety and risk management agenda. The purpose of the directorate was to ensure that patients and clients of the health services in Ireland received the best possible health and personal social care within available resources. The directorate was responsible for implementing the HSE's quality, safety and risk management framework.[85]

In January 2009 the HSE produced a working paper[86] which set out the context, purpose, structure and functions of the new directorate. The working paper noted that the regulatory context in which healthcare is delivered in Ireland has changed radically in recent years. The HSRP of recent years had seen the establishment of HIQA, which regulates healthcare providers – including the HSE – and the Mental Health Commission (MHC), which is also an external regulator of the care of mental health services. The working paper anticipated that the Irish health system would become increasingly regulated in patient safety by international authorities, including the European Union (EU), which had already defined standards in areas such as blood safety.

The working paper defined three key functions of the QCCD. These are referred to as the SEA model: Specify, Enable and Assure. The directorate was expected in the first instance to *specify* or determine standards for care quality, safety and risk management, together with related key performance indicators for the entire organisation – i.e. health and personal social services. It also had an *enabling* function in building capacity to deliver on the quality, safety and risk management agenda by providing support, documented guidance, education, training and direct assistance to enable local service providers to improve the safety and quality of care provided to patients/service users. Finally, the directorate provided *assurance* to the CEO of the HSE by monitoring compliance with key health and personal social services standards and performance against clinical and non-clinical indicators. These assurances were required to be capable of demonstrating to internal and external stakeholders that the best possible health and personal social care outcomes were being achieved for patients/service users within available resources. Ultimately, the directorate was responsible for ensuring that the HSE had the capacity to operate effectively in the new context of increased external regulation (e.g. by HIQA or the MHC) and the requirement for the licensing of providers of health and personal social services.

The initial implementation of the work of the directorate was guided by a number of key operating principles. These included the importance of placing the patient at the centre of the work at all times; the need to pursue actions that can demonstrably improve organisational efficiency and effectiveness evidenced by improved access to and quality of services delivered to patients; the importance of combining central policy and strategy determination with the empowerment of local actors; simplicity and timeliness in all interventions aimed at improving services; and the importance of ensuring that everything that is done can be measured, is achievable, is regularly monitored and is evaluated.

With these basic operational principles in mind, it became apparent that there was a need to identify clear, measurable and time-framed objectives for the work of the directorate. It was agreed that the initial work should centre on issues of access, quality, economy and efficiency. This required the development of a methodology that focused on specific programmes – initiatives in clearly defined areas – to be developed in line with these parameters. This represented the emergence of a series of national clinical programmes[87] that were to become a key part of the healthcare reform process.

The emerging focus for these early initiatives included policy areas such as targeted quality interventions (e.g. surgical check lists); intelligent support materials (e.g. documentation for frameworks, standards, guidelines, standard operating procedures and care pathways) capable of being used at the point of care by patients and clinicians; the development of intelligent care pathways (defined as a pathway whereby the patient can access the right person and/ or information at the right time and for the full spectrum of their journey); and intelligent resource planning by clinicians.

The directorate identified a number of areas of service focus for early initiatives and from these the programmes were identified. These concentrated on specific diseases and treatments, such as stroke (24/7 care, transient ischaemic attacks, use of anticoagulants, stroke units and thrombolysis); cardiovascular disease (heart failure, arrhythmias, blood pressure/lipids and acute coronary syndrome); diabetes mellitus; chronic obstructive pulmonary disease (COPD)/ asthma; epilepsy; depression (transfer of skills, reduced medication and hospital admissions); elective surgical activity (increased activity, reduction in length of hospital stay and elimination of waiting times); and acute medicine. These programmes were to be charged with delivering significant gains in access, quality and cost effectiveness.

In the HSE's 2011 National Service Plan,[88] the national clinical programmes are identified as fundamentally driving the HSE's future thinking as to how clinical services should be delivered. Given their central importance, therefore, it was decided that the management of the national clinical programmes should be separated from the broader role of managing the QCCD in the area of risk and quality in clinical care, with a separate national director appointed to each task. The 2012 National Service Plan[89] identifies the need, as outlined in the national clinical programmes,[90] to move to models of care across all services/care groups which treat patients at the lowest level of complexity and provide services at the lowest possible unit cost.

Programme for Government 2011–2016

On 6 March 2011 the newly elected coalition Government of Fine Gael and Labour finalised their Programme for Government, naming it *Government for National Recovery 2011–2016*.[91] The new Government changed the name of the Department of Health and Children to the Department of Health[92] and the Minister responsible for the Department was now to be known as the Minister for Health. Legal effect was given to this change in SI No 219/2011 – Health and Children (Alteration of Name of Department and Title of Minister) Order 2011, which was signed on 10 May 2011 and came into effect on 4 June 2011. This reversed a change in the name of the department that had been introduced by the Government in 1997, when the name of the department was changed to the Department of Health and Children.

The Programme for Government included an ambitious set of targets for Irish healthcare. The overarching objective was to develop a universal, single-tier health service, bringing to an end what was described in the Programme as the unfair, unequal and inefficient two-tier health system. The outworking of this objective implied that access to medical care should be guaranteed and should be based on need, not income. The model of healthcare delivery would be reformed, moving towards delivering more care in the community.

The Programme set out important reforms of the healthcare system that rowed back many of the changes that had taken place under previous governments. Responsibility for health policy and for the implementation of healthcare reform under the Programme for Government reverted to a centralised model, with the Minister for Health assuming total control of policy and spending. It also proposed that the HSE would cease to exist over time and its functions would return to the Minister for Health and his department or be taken over by the new universal health insurance system that would be introduced, with staff being redeployed accordingly. The HSE hospital purchasing arm would merge with the National Treatment Purchasing Fund (NTPF) to become a new purchaser of public patient care during this period of transition. HSE hospitals would become autonomous providers of care. A Patient Safety Authority, incorporating HIQA, would be established and a special delivery unit (SDU) would be established in the Department of Health.

In keeping with the renewed emphasis on control of public expenditure, the Programme for Government also emphasised the need for ongoing cost control. Reference pricing and greater use of generic medication would be introduced to reduce the State's large drugs bill and the cost to individuals of their medications. Under the new GP contract, the rate of remuneration of GPs would be reduced. Under a new consultants' contract, hospital consultants' remuneration would be reduced. Action would be taken to reduce the cost of procurement for medical equipment and construction of facilities.

The Programme stated that health capital spending would be a priority. Within the health capital budget, the immediate priority areas would be primary care centres, step-down and long-term care facilities and community care facilities such as day centres for older people. The completion and commissioning of the cystic fibrosis unit would be expedited. The National Children's Hospital would be built.

The most novel idea in the Programme for Government was the proposal to introduce a new way of financing the health system. In order to finance the single-tier healthcare service, the Government proposed to introduce universal health insurance (UHI). As a precursor to this, a system of risk equalisation would be introduced for the current insurance market. The system of UHI would be introduced by 2016, with the legislative and organisational groundwork for the system completed within the Government's term of office. UHI would provide guaranteed access to care for all in public and private hospitals on the same basis as private insurance. Insurance with a public or private insurer would be compulsory, with insurance payments related to ability to pay. The State would pay insurance premiums for people on low incomes and subsidise premiums for people on middle incomes. Everyone would have a choice between competing insurers. The voluntary health insurance body, VHI Healthcare, would be kept in public ownership to retain a public option in the UHI system. Exchequer funding for hospital care would go into a Hospital Insurance Fund, which would subsidise or pay insurance premiums for those who qualify for subsidy.

The Hospital Insurance Fund would oversee a strong and reformed system of community rating and risk equalisation; provide direct payments to hospitals for services that are not covered by insurance, such as EDs and ambulances; and provide matching payment to hospitals for treatments delivered. The Hospital Insurance Fund would also control those healthcare costs for which central control is most effective. Under UHI, insurers would be obliged to offer the same package of services to all. This guaranteed UHI package would be determined by the Minister for Health in consultation with the Hospital Insurance Fund and medical experts and would be regularly reviewed under a process to be established in legislation. Insurers would not be allowed to sell insurance giving faster access to procedures covered by the UHI package. Hospitals and clinics which participate in supplying care under UHI would not be allowed to sell faster access to procedures covered by the UHI package. A White Paper on financing UHI would be published early in the Government's first term and would review cost-effective pricing and funding mechanisms for care to be covered under UHI. The legislative basis for UHI would be established by a Universal Health Insurance Act.

On 24 February 2012[93] the Minister for Health established an implementation group on universal health insurance to support the Government to deliver on its commitment to introduce a single-tier health system supported by universal health insurance. It is tasked with developing detailed implementation plans for universal health insurance and with actively driving implementation of various elements of the Government's health reform programme. The group comprises senior civil servants and a mix of individuals with executive responsibilities within the health services and external experts.

The implementation of UHI has significant implications for primary care. It will bring with it the introduction of universal primary care, which will remove fees for GP care. This is to be introduced within the Government's term of office. The legislative basis for universal primary care will be established under a Universal Primary Care Act. Universal primary care will be introduced in phases, so that additional doctors, nurses and other primary care professionals can be recruited. During the term of the Government, GP training places will be increased. GPs will be encouraged to defer retirement, others will be recruited from abroad and the number of practice nurses will be increased so that GPs can delegate care, when appropriate, to nurses.

Access to primary care without fees will be extended in the first year to claimants of free drugs under the Long-Term Illness Scheme at a cost of €17 million. Access to primary care without fees will be extended in the second year to claimants of free drugs under the High-Tech Drugs Scheme at a cost of €15 million. Access to subsidised care will be extended to all in the next phase. Access to care without fees will be extended to all in the final phase. Under universal primary care, GPs will be paid primarily by capitation for the care of their patients and will work in primary care teams with other primary care professionals.

A new GP contract will provide incentives to GPs to care more intensively for patients with chronic illnesses. This will significantly reduce pressures and demands on the hospital system. Registration with a primary care team will be compulsory once the universal primary care system is fully implemented. Exchequer funding for primary care will go to a Primary Care Fund on a transitional basis, which will pay providers of primary care. The goal under UHI will be to create an integrated system of primary and hospital care.

UHI also has significant implications for acute care. It brings with it the concept of universal hospital care. Under UHI, public hospitals will no longer be managed by the HSE. They will be independent, not-for-profit trusts with managers accountable to their boards, which will include representatives of local communities and staff. Smaller hospitals may combine in a local hospital network with a shared management and board. Hospitals will be paid according to the care they deliver and will be incentivised to deliver more care in a 'money follows the patient' system. Insurers will negotiate directly with hospitals to help control costs and encourage innovation in the delivery of care. Insurers will not take over the running of hospitals, which will be independent providers of care separate from insurers as purchasers of care. The Minister for Health will be responsible for hospitals policy and determining that hospitals which play an important role in an area should not be allowed to close under UHI. The Hospital Insurance Fund will assist hospitals in more remote locations that may not have a large throughput of patients to continue to provide important local services. To ensure that hospitals compete on an equal footing, public hospitals will be compensated for costs they bear that private hospitals do not, such as EDs and training healthcare professionals. The Patient Safety

Authority will introduce a national licensing system for hospitals and will oversee the transition of hospitals from the HSE to independent local control. The existing policy of co-location of private hospitals on public hospital lands will cease, as will tax incentives for private hospital developments.

The pathway to the introduction of Universal Health Care Insurance is described in the Programme for Government as: comprising the enactment of the legislative basis for UHI; giving autonomy from the HSE to public hospitals; giving the HSE's function of purchasing care for uninsured patients to a Hospital Care Purchase Agency, which will combine with the National Treatment Purchase Fund (NTPF) to purchase care for the uninsured over the transition period; and separating purchaser-provider functions in order to facilitate the introduction of the 'money follows the patient' system of purchase of care for people without insurance before the implementation of the UHI system.

Another feature in the Programme for Government was the proposal to establish the SDU in the Department of Health to assist the Minister in reducing waiting lists and introducing a major upgrade in the information technology (IT) capabilities of the health system. The unit was established in June 2011[94] with the announcement of the engagement of a senior clinical adviser and it became fully operational in September 2011 with the appointment of a chief operating officer. The development of the unit is portrayed as a key part of plans to radically reform the health system in Ireland. The priorities encompass waiting times for unscheduled and scheduled care and the introduction of a major upgrade in the performance capabilities of the Irish health system. The immediate priorities for the unit were identified as reducing waiting times in emergency departments, which were described as unacceptably high in a number of hospitals; reducing inpatient waiting times, with an instruction from the Minister that public hospitals should have no patients waiting more than twelve months by the end of 2011, reducing to nine months by the end of 2012; reducing outpatient waiting times, as the time from GP referral to an appointment with a consultant was seen as unacceptably long in many specialities; and improving access to diagnostics, as this forms an essential part of the patient journey for all areas of access.

The NTPF is an independent statutory agency established in 2002 with the primary aim of overseeing the faster access to elective hospital-based treatment for public patients. In its Annual Report for 2010,[95] the NTPF describes its mission as 'to reduce the length of time that patients are on hospital waiting lists by offering choice in obtaining access to treatment promptly, safely and to a high standard of patient satisfaction'. The Government has determined that the NTPF capability will be a core part of the SDU's performance management role in holding public hospitals to account. In July 2011,[96] the Minister for Health announced changes in the role of the NTPF to support the SDU. These changes are another stage in the implementation of the Government's health reform agenda and follow on from the establishment of the SDU. In December 2011,[97] the chief operations officer of the SDU assumed responsibility for the management of the NTPF. The main changes are that the NTPF will target particular backlogs, rather than routinely accepting referrals of patients waiting over three months, and the requirement that the NTPF purchase 90 per cent of treatments in the private sector is ended.

There is evidence of some early success for the work of the SDU and the NTPF.[98] In the area of unscheduled care in emergency departments (EDs), the cumulative number waiting on trolleys at 8.00 a.m. across the country for the first sixteen days of January 2012 was 5,046. This compares with 6,893 during the same period in 2011, a reduction of 27 per cent. In the area of scheduled care (surgery and outpatients), at the end of 2011 approximately 95 per cent (41 hospitals) met the target to eliminate those waiting over twelve months from their active list. This compares to 28 hospitals at the end of 2010 that had patients waiting over twelve months for treatment on the active list. The improvements are impressive, especially against a backdrop of a reduction in funding of almost €1 billion for the health services in 2011 as part of the overall programme of reduction in public expenditure agreed as part of the IMF–ECB–EC bailout package.

The SDU set a number of ambitious targets for 2012. Among these are to ensure that 95 per cent of all attendees at EDs are discharged or admitted within six hours of registration, and that those who need to be admitted through the ED wait no more than nine hours from registration; to ensure that nobody is waiting more than nine months for planned surgery; and to set and implement targets for improved access to outpatient and diagnostic services in the first quarter of 2012.

The Programme for Government also contained a number of statements of intent in relation to the care of older people and community care. It stated that investment in the supply of more and better care for older people in the community and in residential settings would be a priority and that additional funding would be provided each year for the care of older people. It was intended that this funding should go to more residential places, more home care packages and the delivery of more home help and other professional community care services. The Fair Deal system of financing nursing home care, introduced during the lifetime of the previous Government, which provided for a charge against the estate of older persons to finance long-term care, would be reviewed with a view to developing a secure and equitable system of financing for community and long-term care which supported older people to stay in their own homes.

The Government is also committed to a continued emphasis on integrated care, which had been a principal theme of the previous Government's health policy. This is based on the principle that the integration of care in all settings is key to efficient healthcare delivery, in which the right care is delivered in the right place. Integration of care would be the responsibility of an integrated care agency under the aegis of the Minister for Health, which would oversee the flow of centrally tax-funded resources between the different arms of the system so that there would be incentives for care to occur in the best setting.

In the area of mental health, the Programme for Government incorporates the recommendations of *A Vision for Change: Report of the Expert Group on Mental Health Policy*,[99] the principal strategic policy document introduced by the previous Government. The Government stated that it was committed to reducing the stigma of mental illness, ensuring early and appropriate intervention and vastly improving access to modern mental health services in the community. It is intended that a comprehensive range of mental health services will be included as part of the standard insurance package offered under UHI. Given the central role of primary care in the proposed reforms, the Government said that it would ensure that patients can access mental health services such as psychologists and counsellors in the primary care setting and that it would strengthen GP education and training in mental health so that they could better diagnose, treat and refer patients as necessary.

The Government plans to ringfence €35 million annually from within the health budget to develop community mental health teams and services, as outlined in *A Vision for Change*, to ensure early access to more appropriate services for adults and children and improved integration with primary care services. Part of the ringfenced funding would be used to implement Reach Out, the national suicide prevention strategy,[100] and reduce the high levels of suicide. It plans to close unsuitable psychiatric institutions, moving patients to more appropriate community-based facilities, and to develop specific strategies for elderly patients and those with intellectual disabilities who remain under the care of the mental health services. The programme also includes a commitment to develop a national Alzheimer's and other dementias strategy by 2013, to increase awareness, ensure early diagnosis and intervention and the development of enhanced community-based services. This strategy will be implemented over five years.

To ensure a joined-up approach to mental health in the community, the Government intends to establish a cross-departmental group to ensure that good mental health is a policy goal across a range of people's life experiences, including education, employment and housing. The Government stated that it would endeavour to end the practice of placing children and adolescents in adult psychiatric wards. Finally, it would review the Mental Health Act 2001[101] in consultation with service users, carers and other stakeholders, informed by human rights standards, and introduce a Mental Capacity Bill[102] in line with the United Nations (UN) Convention on the Rights of Persons with Disabilities.[103] In 2012, the Government published the *Interim Report of the Steering Group on the Review of the Mental Health Act 2001*[104] and the Assisted Decision-Making (Capacity) Bill 2012.[105] These will be discussed in more detail in Chapter 6.

In December 2011[106] the Government approved the drafting of legislation involving significant changes in the governance in the HSE. The legislation, once implemented, will replace the current board/chief executive structure with a Directorate (or transitional governance) structure. The putting in place of a new Directorate structure in the HSE is a key component in the move towards UHI. Legislation that will have the cumulative effect of abolishing the HSE will be brought forward on a sequential basis, as part of the overall health reform programme, with functions transferring elsewhere as part of the move towards a system of UHI.

This fundamental alteration of the operation of the health services will involve a separation of the purchasing of health and social services from the provision of health and social services. This in turn will allow the implementation of a full 'money follows the patient' system, where providers are paid on the basis of services delivered. In order to achieve a new degree of transparency, accountability and efficiency – prior to its abolition – the HSE will be reorganised along service lines. The new Directorate structure identifies clear areas of priority and the appointment of directors for those service lines. Seven areas of service provision have been identified and these will be organised within the Directorate structure. The seven areas are hospital care, primary care, mental health, children and family services, social care, public health, and corporate/shared services.

Seven directors are to be appointed:[107] one of them will be the Director General. The Minister for Health will determine the precise functions of the directors. The Minister will bring forward detailed proposals at a later date for the reorganisation of the HSE at the Directorate, regional and local level in a manner that facilitates a smooth transition from the current structure to the structures required under UHI. On 29 May 2012 the Government approved the Heads of a Bill that will see the formal abolition of the Board of the HSE and the establishment of the Directorate structure.[108]

The purpose of this Directorate team will be twofold: to run the health services as they exist and to prepare for the transformation required in the move to UHI. It is intended that the identification of the seven service lines will provide clarity in relation to the delivery of the relevant services under the responsibility of the directors and greater financial transparency and accountability in assessing those services. With the passing of the legislation, the Minister for Health will provide a clear statement on the precise timeline for further reform in the run-up to UHI. A White Paper setting out how UHI will be implemented is to be published before the end of 2012.

The Government also announced that the Primary Care Fund, as provided for in the Programme for Government, will be established as a matter of priority. Its early establishment will support the roll-out of free GP care, beginning in 2012. The Integrated Care Agency and the Hospital Care Purchase Agency, which are likewise provided for in the Programme for Government, will also be established during 2012.

In March 2012[109] the Minister published a new policy direction for the establishment of public hospital groups. Hospitals will be organised in groups throughout the country. A group chief executive will be appointed, responsible for organising services in an optimum way across a number of hospitals. The Minister wrote to the HSE outlining his policy on setting up the hospital groups, and on the management arrangements for those groups, as part of a series of steps to implement the Government's health reform agenda. The new initiative has involved the Minister setting out his policy under section 10 of the Health Act 2004,[110] which allows the Minister to give formal policy direction to the HSE. The Minister signalled his intention to use this function afforded to him by the Act to set out the direction of policy to the HSE. Work on developing the new hospital groups is under way and there will be appropriate consultation before the Government makes decisions. In particular, the Minister intends to publish a framework for the development of smaller hospitals.

In January 2012[111] the Minister announced that the national clinical programmes would move to the Department of Health. These clinical programmes were developed by the QCCD created within the HSE in 2009.[112] The directorate, under the leadership of a national director for quality care, created 26 programmes in key healthcare areas: acute coronary syndrome (ACS); acute medicine; asthma; audiology; blood transfusion; care of the elderly; COPD; critical care; dermatology; diabetes; elective surgery (ESP); emergency medicine (EMP); epilepsy; heart failure; medicines management and pharmacotherapeutic interventions; obstetrics and gynaecology; outpatient parenteral antimicrobial therapy (OPAT); orthopaedics; palliative care; prevention of healthcare-associated infection (HCAI) and antimicrobial resistance (AMR); primary care; radiology; rehabilitation medicine; renal; rheumatology; and stroke.

Each of these programmes sets a number of clear, attainable and measurable objectives and an interdisciplinary team of clinicians and managers will roll out a programme of quality improvement and efficiency on a national basis. The moving of these programmes back to the Department of Health is a logical consequence of the Government's decision to return responsibility for policy, spending and implementation of healthcare services to the Department. The programmes will also be working in close harmony with the SDU in improving performance across the system. The national cancer control programme, which has operated independently of the national clinical programmes and which has seen significant improvements in cancer outcomes, will also be located in the Department of Health.

Finally, a new programme management office will be established in the Department of Health to ensure the wide-ranging process of reform is implemented.

In July 2012 the Minister published the Health Service Executive (Governance) Bill 2012.[113] The purpose of the Bill was to abolish the board structure of the HSE and provide for a Directorate to be the new governing body for the HSE in place of the board.[114] The Directorate would be headed up by a Director General. The Bill also included provisions for further accountability arrangements for the HSE and a number of technical amendments to take account of the replacement of the board structure by the Directorate structure. The Bill was intended to make the HSE more directly accountable. Under the provisions of the Bill, the Directorate will consist of a Director General and a number of directors. In anticipation of the legislative changes, the Minister directed the HSE to recruit and appoint heads of a number of services, including health and well-being, hospitals, primary care, mental health, and social care. The persons appointed as heads of these services will, together with the head of children's services, be appointed as members of the Directorate. On 27 July 2012 the Minister announced the appointment of a new Director General for the HSE.[115]

Under the provisions of the Bill, the Directorate would be accountable to the Minister for the performance of the HSE's functions as well as its own. As chairperson of the Directorate, the Director General would account to the Minister, through the Secretary General of the Department of Health, on the performance of the HSE's functions. The Bill allows the Minister to issue directions to the HSE on the implementation of Ministerial and Government policies and objectives. The Minister is also empowered to specify priorities for the HSE which must be taken into account in the preparation of the service plan.[116]

The Directorate is a transitional, interim arrangement as part of a move towards the implementation of the Government's health reform programme. As the health reform programme advances, it is intended that the HSE should no longer exist. The sequence of events and the timeline intended to lead to the abolition of the HSE were outlined by the Department of Health[117] as follows:

- Fourth quarter of 2012 – establishment of the new Directorate
- 1 January 2013 – Voted expenditure returns to the Department of Health

- 2013 – New hospital groups introduced and reform of the integrated service areas
- 2013 – New funding systems introduced, e.g. Primary Care Fund
- 2014 – Creation of the new Integrated Care Agency that will replace the HSE

A formal endorsement of the Programme for Government as the cornerstone of health policy for the foreseeable future is contained in the *Department of Health Statement of Strategy 2011–2014*,[118] which was published on 8 May 2012.[119] The strategy sets out the aims of the Department of Health for the period up to and including 2014. During that time, it is envisaged that the provision of health services will be radically reshaped, in line with the commitments contained in the Programme for Government. The strategy states that the purpose of the health service in Ireland is to improve the health and well-being of the people. The role of the Department of Health is to provide strategic leadership for the health service and ensure that Government policies for the sector are translated into actions and implemented effectively. In launching the strategy, the Minister for Health emphasised that over the period there would be a move towards a health system that would provide access based on need rather than income, underpinned by a strengthened primary care sector, a restructured hospital sector and a more transparent 'money follows the patient' system of funding. The Minister said that this must be done against the backdrop of economic and fiscal conditions that were the most challenging in the history of the State.

CHAPTER 3

The Professions of Nursing and Midwifery

The Statutory Basis of the Professions

The development of a statute-based system of self-regulation that requires nurses and midwives to be eligible for inclusion on a register provides the basis for the characterisation of nursing and midwifery as professions. At a single stroke, the Nurses Registration Act 1919[120] provided nursing and midwifery with a statutory basis and established a register of general nurses. The Nurses Acts of 1950, 1961 and 1985[121] retained this register and formalised the authority under which general nurses could practise.

Nursing and midwifery have evolved as professions over the years in response to developments in the health services and developments within the professions themselves, culminating most recently in a radical review of the roles of nursing and midwifery by the Commission on Nursing in 1998.[122] The findings and recommendations of the Commission had profound implications for the development of the professions and for the roles of nurses and midwives in the health services. It has resulted in the introduction of a number of significant changes in the professions, in particular the introduction of a clinical career pathway developed by the National Council for the Professional Development of Nursing and Midwifery.

Developments over the years since the Commission completed its work have included the emergence of an increased number of nurse-/midwife-led services, the involvement of nurses and midwives in prescribing, and major changes in the demands being placed on nurse and midwife managers. There has also been a radical transformation in the provision of educational opportunities for nurses and midwives, at both pre- and post-registration levels, including increased professional development opportunities.

The *Report of the Commission on Nursing* made a number of recommendations in relation to the professions, some of which it identified as being urgent. One of these was the introduction of legislation amending the Nurses Act 1985,[123] in order to place the safety of the public at the centre of professional regulation for nursing and midwifery. The Commission recommended that this amendment should be put before the Oireachtas by early 1999. Twelve years later, the recommendation was eventually implemented. At the end of 2011, the Nurses Act 1985 was replaced by the Nurses and Midwives Act 2011.[124] The Act brought to an end a period of self-regulation for the professions that had stretched from the first Act in 1919 to the end of 2011. It represented a radical overhaul in the way in which nursing and midwifery are regulated, with a new emphasis on public safety and accountability and the introduction of a lay majority board.

The Nurses and Midwives Act 2011

The Nurses and Midwives Act 2011 was signed into legislation on 21 December 2011. The Commencement Order (SI No 715 of 2011)[125] in respect of sections 1 and 2 (repealing the Nurses Act 1985 and providing for the establishment of the Nursing and Midwifery Board of Ireland) and part 12 (providing for the dissolution of the National Council) of the Nurses and Midwives Act 2011 was signed by the Minister for Health and took effect from midnight of 31 December 2011.

The provisions of the Nurses and Midwives Act 2011 are broadly in line with the provisions of the Medical Practitioners Act 2007[126] and the Health and Social Care Professionals Act 2005.[127]

A paper[128] drafted by the Department of Health and Children in 2010 noted that the Minister for Health and Children was committed to the introduction of new primary legislation for the regulation of nurses and midwives as part of the wider reforms of the health services and the modernisation of the regulation of all healthcare professionals. The 2011 Act is reflective of a significant change within the health services in Ireland that places public safety at the heart of the regulation of health professions. Subsequent health strategies, in particular *Quality and Fairness: A Health System for You,*[129] emphasised the importance of equality, fairness, access and patient centredness, all key elements of public and patient safety. *Building a Culture of Patient Safety: Report of the Commission on Patient Safety and Quality Assurance*[130] further emphasised the need for healthcare professionals to place the safety and welfare of their patients at the centre of their professional structures of governance and accountability.

Until 2011, the Nurses Act 1985[131] provided the statutory framework for the regulation of the professions of nursing and midwifery. It provided for the establishment of An Bord Altranais to oversee the regulation of the profession. The provision of health services both within Ireland and internationally has moved on considerably since the Nurses Act 1985 was signed into law. Patient safety has become the defining feature in the regulation of healthcare professions. New developments since the 1985 Act include significant progress in the practices of nursing and midwifery, advances in education and training, the recognition of midwifery as a distinct profession, an increased emphasis on accountability, the importance of the rights of the patient and the reform of and changes within the health system in Ireland, as well as changes at EU level.[132]

Government and key stakeholders increasingly recognised the need to modernise the regulatory framework for all healthcare professionals, to include a greater emphasis on patient safety, governance, accountability, openness and fairness and efficiency of disciplinary procedures and an assurance of standards. The Nurses Act 2011 reflects these requirements and makes provision for a strengthened legislative framework that prioritises public accountability and the safety of the patient/client.

The Act provides for a greater non-nursing/midwifery representation on the board of the regulatory body and enhances arrangements for the maintenance of high standards of practice. Members of the public have in recent years shown a higher level of interest in the provision and quality of care provided by the health services and have highlighted the need to introduce measures to enhance professional performance and to deal more quickly with individuals whose fitness to practise may be in question while also allowing for individual nurses'/midwives' rights to be respected.[133]

The long title of the Act provides a useful summary of the intentions behind the legislation. It contains a list of the objectives and purpose of the Act. In the first instance, the Act is introduced for the purpose of the enhancement of the protection of the public in its dealings with nurses and midwives. In order to provide for that, the Act makes provisions for the establishment of a board to be known as An Bord Altranais agus Cnáimhseachais na hÉireann, or, in English, the Nursing and Midwifery Board of Ireland. The Act also gives legal effect to the recognition of midwifery as a distinct profession that had been signalled by the *Report of the Commission on Nursing*.[134] The key provisions of the Act relate to the registration, regulation and control of nurses and midwives; the enhancement of the high standards of professional education, training and competence of nurses and midwives; and the investigation of complaints against nurses and midwives. By changing the composition of board membership and the introduction of a number of new governance procedures, the Act increases the public accountability of the Board. The Act also provides for the dissolution of the National Council for the Professional Development of Nursing and Midwifery and repeals the Nurses Act 1985.

The regulation of nurses and midwives in Ireland is now be the responsibility of a regulatory body known as the Nursing and Midwifery Board of Ireland (the Board), whose primary responsibility will be the protection of the public in their dealings with nurses and midwives; for the first time, it will have a lay majority board. This, in effect, means that the professions are no longer self-regulated. The Act also provides for the Board to submit to the Minister a statement of its strategy, i.e. its corporate and business plans, and a report on its accounts and its performance against its strategy. The Minister reserves the right to request amendments to the proposed strategy of the Board. The Act, therefore, is a key component in the construction of a system of governance and accountability for the health services of Ireland that places public interest and patient safety at the centre.

The Act also introduces measures to ensure that the integrity of the practice of nursing and midwifery is protected. The public needs to be assured that any person who uses the title 'nurse' or 'midwife' is entitled to do so because of his or her professional competence. The requirement for everyone who wishes to practise as a nurse or midwife to register with the Board is an essential part of that guarantee. It also prohibits anyone who is not registered from using the title 'nurse' or 'midwife'. The register must also identify those who are candidates for the professions during the course of their professional education and training. Systems of professional registration are essential components in the system of governance and accountability. They are there to protect the integrity of the professions and the use of the titles associated with nursing and midwifery practice.

The Act emphasises the importance of maintaining and developing high standards of professional education and training for nurses and midwives. Nursing and midwifery in Ireland has come a long way from the days of the apprenticeship model of training. Today, Irish nurses and midwives enjoy a degree-based system of education in third-level institutions with close links to clinical settings. Considerable investment in the education of nurses and midwives has taken place over the last ten years. As a result, great progress has been made in providing the professions with a stronger theoretical and research base. This has resulted in a stronger sense of professional identity. The quality and relevance of these education and training programmes is essential if nursing and midwifery is to fulfil its role. The Act provides for the ongoing development of standards for nurse and midwifery education and the accreditation of programmes of education necessary for the purposes of registration. The definition of standards also applies to post-registration education and training courses, particularly where nurses and midwives are moving into areas of specialist or advanced practice.

The Act outlines the respective duties of the HSE and the Board in relation to the education and training of nurses and midwives.[135] It is the duty of the HSE to facilitate the education and training of candidates for the professions. In relation to specialist nursing and midwifery education and training, the HSE's role is expressed as one of promoting and coordinating in cooperation with the Board and the training bodies approved by the Board. It also has a role in workforce planning in order to meet the specialist nursing and midwifery requirements of the service. The HSE also has a broad role of advising the Minister, after consultation with the nursing and midwifery training bodies, the Higher Education Authority and others on nursing and midwifery education and training and on all other matters, including financial matters, relating to the development and coordination of specialist nursing and midwifery education and training. It is the duty of the Board to set and publish in the prescribed manner the standards of nursing and midwifery education and training for first-time registration and post-registration specialist nursing and midwifery qualifications and to monitor adherence to these standards.

The provisions of the Act in relation to specialisation in nursing and midwifery place responsibility on the HSE for the identification of the needs of the services in this area and promotion and development of specialist nursing and midwifery opportunities. It is the role of the Board to ensure that proper standards, criteria and guidelines are in place to ensure that, as these roles develop, they are compliant with agreed standards. Pending commencement orders for the implementation of the provisions of the legislation, the standards and criteria that apply to specialist nursing and midwifery are those that were defined by the National Council.

The Act makes provision for the maintenance and assurance of professional competence of registered nurses and midwives. It is the responsibility of each nurse and midwife to maintain his or her own competence. However, the Act provides for the definition of new models and frameworks whereby this can be monitored and assured. Employers have a role in facilitating the involvement of their professional staff in activities designed specifically to maintain and enhance professional competence. A robust system of governance aimed at the protection of the public will include systems for the monitoring and audit of activity in the area of maintenance of competence. Competence assurance provides great opportunities for nurses and midwives to engage in meaningful continuing professional development processes related to their clinical practice. Professional development processes may include the maintenance of portfolios, engagement in clinical supervision, supervised clinical practice and clinical audit to support demonstration of competency development and attainment. Competence assurance should ultimately lead to enhanced clinical effectiveness and improved population health.

Nursing and midwifery practice must adhere to the highest standards of professional conduct. A robust code of professional conduct based on defined standards of practice is an essential ingredient of good governance and accountability. The Act charges the Board with providing the professions with clear guidance in this area and promoting throughout the profession a commitment to the highest standards of professional conduct. Increasingly, in a modern health service, professional practice takes place in a multidisciplinary environment, involving close cooperation with other clinical and non-clinical professional staff. The introduction of the clinical directorate model for the organisation of health service delivery is built on the principles of multidisciplinary cooperation in service delivery teams. Nurses and midwives have a key role to play in these teams and they need clear guidance on how they can develop their practice in this environment in a manner that ensures the highest standards of public safety and the most effective cooperation with other healthcare professionals. Nurses and midwives should be able to look to their regulatory body for this kind of guidance, including guidance on scope of practice and standards of professional conduct.

Efficient and effective systems are needed to deal with complaints and to assess fitness to practise. Complaints against individual nurses and midwives should be handled in a fair, open, transparent and efficient manner. The Act provides for preliminary assessment of complaints prior to challenges regarding fitness to practise. This should reduce the number of fitness to practise hearings and provide a cost-effective and efficient mechanism for dealing with complaints. When a full fitness to practise hearing is required, these should be held, as far as possible, in public. In keeping with the principle of the pre-eminence of public safety in professional regulation, members of the fitness to practise and complaints panels will include a majority of lay persons.

Role of the Board

Part 2, article 8 of the Nurses and Midwives Act 2011 sets out clearly the overall role of the Board and article 9 outlines its key functions.

The objective of the Board is described as the protection of the public in its dealing with nurses and midwives and the integrity of the practice of nursing and midwifery through the promotion of high standards of professional education, training and practice and professional conduct among nurses and midwives.

The principal functions of the Board include the establishment and maintenance of the register of nurses and midwives and a candidate register for nursing and midwifery students. It is also responsible for the establishment of procedures and criteria for assessment and registration in the register for both qualified nurses/midwives and candidates. The Board must also establish the divisions of the register and issue certificates of registration and renewal of registration.

One of the key roles of the Board is the definition of standards for the education of nurses and midwives. It is responsible for the approval of programmes of education and further education necessary for the purposes of registration and continued registration and for keeping these programmes under review.

The Board is designated to act as the competent authority for the purposes of the mutual recognition of professional qualifications of nurses and midwives awarded in or recognised by member states of the European Union or other relevant states within the meaning of the Regulations of 2008,[136] and all matters referred to in Directive 2005/36/EC.[137] This European Directive relates to the role of a competent authority for the purposes of the recognition of professional qualifications of nurses and midwives. As the competent authority, the Board is empowered to enter into agreement with the competent authorities in other countries for the mutual recognition of qualifications and authorisations to practise.

The Board is also required to specify standards of practice for registered nurses and registered midwives, including the establishment, publication, maintenance and review of appropriate guidance on all matters related to professional conduct and ethics for registered nurses and registered midwives. It must also provide appropriate guidance on the maintenance of the professional competence of registered nurses and registered midwives and issue a code of professional conduct for registered nurses and registered midwives.

The Board is responsible for a function that was previously fulfilled by the National Council, i.e. the specification of criteria regarding the creation by employers of specialist nursing and midwifery posts. This relates to the creation in clinical settings of specialist nursing and midwifery posts designated as clinical nurse/midwife specialists (CNS/CMS) and advanced nurse/midwife practitioners (ANP/AMP).

Prior to the introduction of the Nurses and Midwives Act 2011, it was the function of the National Council to support the creation of specialist and advanced practice posts and provide clear frameworks for approval/accreditation of these posts.[138] This kind of regulation of advanced practice has been described in research[139] in the United Kingdom as essential. This is not universally accepted in other countries[140] and the lack of such regulation can lead to role confusion[141] and uncertainty about how the roles of clinical specialists and advanced practitioners differ.[142] Confusion is evidenced by a proliferation of terms such as 'nurse practitioner', 'nurse consultant',[143] 'advanced practice nurse' and the more common 'clinical nurse specialist'.[144] With the abolition of the National Council by the Nurses and Midwives Act 2011, the responsibility for providing this kind of regulation falls on the Board. The responsibility for the development of the posts and encouraging individuals to take up the roles lies with the HSE. This division of responsibility could potentially lead to a reduction in leadership in this important area.

The Board is also responsible for the establishment of committees to enquire into complaints about nurses and midwives and to make decisions and give directions under part 9 of the Act (Reports of Fitness to Practise Committees) relating to the imposition of sanctions on registered nurses and registered midwives.

As part of its duty to protect the public, the Board must advise the public on all matters of general interest relating to the functions of the Board, its area of expertise and other matters of interest to the public relating to nurses and midwives and their practice, including public advertisement of the objectives, functions and contact details of the Board from time to time.

In general, the Board is required to advise the Minister, either at the Minister's request or on its own initiative, on all matters relating to the other functions conferred on it by any provision of the Act, and perform any other function conferred on it under any other provision of this Act or of any other enactment.

The principal instrument used by the Board in the fulfilment of its functions is the capacity to make rules. Part 2, section 13 of the Act confers on the Board the authority to make rules 'for the purposes of the better operation of any provision of this Act'. The most recent version of these rules is the *Nurses Rules 2010*,[145] made under the provisions of the Nurses Act 1985. In addition to these rules, the Board will also issue guidance notes for nurses and midwives and for the public.[146] These guidelines include a code of conduct for nurses and midwives, practice standards and guidelines for nurses and midwives and guidance for education providers in relation to the standards that should apply to the development of curricula for nurse and midwife education programmes.

The Act also makes provision for a change to the membership of the Board. Under the Nurses Act 1985, membership of the board of An Bord Altranais consisted of twenty-nine persons: seventeen of these were nurses from education, management and clinical practice and twelve were appointed by the Minister. Of the twelve ministerial appointments, one was a nurse, nine were representative of healthcare management and the Department of Health and two were to be 'persons representative of the interest of the general public'.[147] Thus, nurses and midwives made up a majority on the membership of the board of An Bord Altranais and, in this sense, the regulation of the professions was truly 'self-regulation'.

With the change in emphasis in the Nurses and Midwives Act 2011 to protection of the public and accountability, the composition of the membership of the Board has been changed completely. Part 4, section 22 outlines the membership of the Board. It will consist of twenty-three persons: eleven of these will be nurses or midwives, covering the areas of education, nursing management, each of the branches of the register and care of older persons (eight of the eleven nurses are to be elected by members of the professions, the other three will be appointed by the Minister from lists provided by the HSE and educational establishments); the additional twelve members will not be nurses or midwives and will include representatives of the medical profession, the health and social care professions, public and voluntary healthcare management, education and five members of the public appointed by the Minister. This lay majority on the Board is to be replicated in all of the committees of the Board, including, most importantly, the fitness to practise committee.

On 25 July 2012 the Commencement Order (SI No 275 of 2012)[148] in respect of section 22 (relating to membership of the Board, nominations by the Minister and provisions for the election of members of the Board) was signed by the Minister. On foot of this, arrangements for the election of members of the Board have been made. Elections take place during the third quarter of 2012.

Meetings of the fitness to practise committee, set up to hear complaints against members of the professions, are to be held in public unless good reasons can be provided as to why they should not be.[149] This is in keeping with the general ethos of the Act, which constantly refers throughout to the public interest, keeping members of the public informed, publication of documentation, making information available to the public and generally adopting a position of openness and transparency in all of its functions. This mirrors similar provisions in other regulatory instruments governing healthcare professions, most notably the Medical Practitioners Act 2007 and the Health and Social Care Professionals Act 2005.

At the time of writing (October 2012), An Bord Altranais continues to operate under the provisions of the Nurses Act 1985 pending commencement orders for the remaining sections of the legislation.

Divisions of the Register

There are a number of divisions of the Register of Nurses maintained by An Bord Altranais. The principal divisions of the register and their respective titles are registered general nurse (RGN), registered midwife (RM), registered psychiatric nurse (RPN), registered nurse intellectual disability (RNID), registered children's nurse (RCN) and registered public health nurse (PHN). In addition, the register contains divisions for registered nurse tutor (RNT), registered nurse prescriber (RNP), advanced nurse practitioner (ANP) and advanced midwife practitioner (AMP).

In 2011 there were 67,130 nurses and midwives on the active register. Nurses and midwives can hold more than one registration and at the end of 2011 there were 89,723 active qualifications registered with An Bord Altranais as outlined in Table 1.[150] At the end of 2011 the Health Service Executive reported that there were 35,993 WTE nursing and midwifery posts.[151] This figure does not include nurses and midwives employed in the private sector. It should also be remembered that there are many nurses and midwives on the active register who are not currently employed in the health services in Ireland.

Table 1: Active Qualifications Registered with An Bord Altranais, 2011[152]

Divisions of the Register	
General Nursing	55,819
Midwifery	12,065
Psychiatric Nursing	9,384
Intellectual Disability Nursing	4,615
Children's Nursing	4,157
Public Health Nursing	2,414
Other Qualifications Registered	
Advanced Midwife Practitioner	4
Advanced Nurse Practitioner	97
Registered Nurse Prescriber	386
Registered Nurse Tutor	600
Other	182
Total	**89,723**

Registered General Nurse

General nurses provide care for patients/clients in a wide variety of settings and within a wide range of complexity. They work with patients with acute and chronic illnesses in both hospital and community settings. They provide care to elderly patients/clients and palliative care for those who are close to death. They also work in emergency departments, operating theatres, intensive care units and many other settings in acute hospital settings. Care provided in hospitals and other healthcare institutions can include long-term care, day-facility care and outpatient care. Increasingly, general nurses are working across the boundaries of acute hospital settings and community care settings, including engaging in outreach programmes as part of integrated care provision – including in patients' homes – following up with discharged patients, and educating and supporting family members and other carers. General nurses are the backbone of the healthcare services: they account for almost two-thirds of the total qualifications on the register. They are the key coordinators of care in most care settings and they take responsibility for care planning and for implementing and monitoring care plans. General nurses are also usually responsible for coordinating the input of other clinical and healthcare professionals.

An Bord Altranais outlines five domains of competence[153] which represent the level that the student of nursing or midwifery must reach on completion of the education programme for entry to the register maintained by An Bord Altranais.[154] Competence is defined as the ability of the registered nurse to practise safely and effectively, fulfilling his/her professional responsibility within his/her scope of practice. The five domains of competence are:

- Professional ethical practice, defined as practising in accordance with legislation that affects nursing practice and practising within the limits of their own competence and taking measures to develop their own competence.
- Holistic approaches to care and the integration of knowledge, defined as conducting a systematic holistic assessment of client needs based on nursing theory and evidence-based practice; planning care in consultation with the client, taking into consideration the therapeutic regimes of all members of the healthcare team; implementing planned nursing care/interventions to

achieve the identified outcomes; evaluating client progress towards expected outcomes; and reviewing plans in accordance with evaluation data and consultation with the client.

- Interpersonal relationships, defined as establishing and maintaining caring therapeutic interpersonal relationships with individuals/clients/groups/communities, collaborating with all members of the healthcare team and documenting relevant information.
- Organisation and management of care, defined as effectively managing the nursing care of individuals/clients/groups/communities, delegating to other nurses activities commensurate with their competence and within their scope of professional practice, and facilitating the coordination of care.
- Personal and professional development, defined as acting to enhance the personal and professional development of self and others.

The aim is to ensure that students acquire the skills of critical analysis, problem-solving, decision-making and reflective skills and abilities essential to the art and science of nursing and midwifery. Safe and effective nursing and midwifery practice requires a sound underpinning of theoretical knowledge that informs practice and is, in turn, informed by that practice. Within complex and changing healthcare environments, it is essential that practice is based on the best available evidence.

Registered Midwife

The accepted international definition of the midwife is the one that has been adopted by the International Confederation of Midwives (ICM), the International Federation of Gynaecology and Obstetrics (FIGO) and the WHO.[155] An Bord Altranais endorses the definition of a midwife as adopted and amended by the ICM in 2005 and 2011,[156] which states:

> A midwife is a person who, having been regularly admitted to a midwifery educational programme, duly recognised in the country in which it is located, has successfully completed the prescribed course of studies in midwifery and has acquired the requisite qualifications to be registered and/or legally licensed to practise midwifery. The midwife is recognised

as a responsible and accountable professional who works in partnership with women to give the necessary support, care and advice during pregnancy, labour and the postpartum period, to conduct births on the midwife's own responsibility and to provide care for the newborn and the infant. This care includes preventative measures, the promotion of normal birth, the detection of complications in mother and child, the accessing of medical care or other appropriate assistance and the carrying out of emergency measures. The midwife has an important task in health counselling and education, not only for the woman, but also within the family and the community. This work should involve antenatal education and preparation for parenthood and may extend to women's health, sexual or reproductive health and child care. A midwife may practise in any setting including home, community, hospitals, clinics or health units.[157]

The *Report of the Commission on Nursing* identified the midwifery profession as being distinct from nursing, and as possessing exclusive skills in relation to maternity care. This was formally recognised and given a statutory basis in the Nurses and Midwives Act 2011.[158] The ICM identifies a number of key midwifery concepts that define the unique role of midwives in promoting the health of women and childbearing families. These include partnership with women to promote self-care and the health of mothers, infants and families; respect for human dignity and for women as persons with full human rights; advocacy for women so that their voices are heard; cultural sensitivity, including working with women and healthcare providers to overcome those cultural practices that harm women and babies; and a focus on health promotion and disease prevention that views pregnancy as a normal life event.

Registered Psychiatric Nurse

An Bord Altranais defines psychiatric nursing as:

A specialist nursing discipline with the primary objectives to facilitate the maximum development of the mental health of the individual who has psychiatric problems and to promote psychiatric nursing. The basis of the work of the psychiatric nurse is the relationship the nurse has with the person and their families who use the mental health services. The manner in which the psychiatric nurse develops this relationship, in partnership with those who use the services and their carers, and the skills the nurse uses within these relationships is the focus of psychiatric nursing.[159]

In 1984 the Department of Health published *The Psychiatric Services: Planning for the Future*.[160] This document signalled a fundamental change in the planning, development and delivery of mental health services in Ireland. In particular, a decision was taken that there should be a shift towards a community mental health service and away from what had up to then been an institution-led service. Delivery of services was to be moved from inpatient services in psychiatric hospitals to specialist units in general hospitals, with an emphasis on rehabilitation and eventual return to the community. Thus, mental health services were to be integrated into mainstream medical care, with a particular emphasis on caring for people within their own communities and their own homes. This policy shift meant a major change in the role of psychiatric nurses and provided a unique opportunity for the development of new skills and roles.[161] The publication in 2006 of the most recent policy review for psychiatric services, *A Vision for Change*,[162] re-emphasised the importance of the community-based dimension of psychiatric care through the promotion of the concept of community mental health teams (CMHTs), consisting of different healthcare professionals providing services within their catchment area.

Registered Nurse Intellectual Disability

The registered nurse intellectual disability provides a range of services across a wide variety of locations, addressing the partic- ular and complex needs of clients, and requiring particular skills and personal qualities distinct from those in other disciplines of nursing. An Bord Altranais describes how intellectual disability nurses provide a specialised form of care that is different from other disciplines of nursing:

> The philosophy of care of a person with an intellectual disabil- ity contains a number of implicit principles, which embrace the concept that all persons with all levels of ability have the same rights and, in so far as possible, the same responsibilities as other members of society. They have a right and a need to

live within the community like other people and they have a right to receive those services necessary to meet their specialised and changing needs. They should receive, if and when necessary, professional assistance and services which will allow recognition, development and expression of the individuality of each person. Nurses who work with persons with an intellectual disability have a diversity of roles, from intensive physical nursing of individuals with profound handicap to supportive guidance in the management and habilitation of children, adolescents and adults. The care of persons with an intellectual disability forms part of the nursing profession as a whole, yet it is specialised and very different from other disciplines of nursing.[163]

The first training schools offering a three-year course in mental handicap nursing opened in 1959. Mental handicap nursing in the early 1960s focused on the treatment and care of the severely disabled of all ages and the treatment, care and training of the lower ranges of moderately disabled children and moderately and mildly disabled adults and of others with mental handicaps.[164] More schools of mental handicap nursing were established from that time until 2002, and the syllabus of training has been revised on several occasions to reflect trends in care and service provision.[165] The *Nurses Rules 2004*[166] replaced the title 'registered mental handicap nurse' with the title 'registered nurse intellectual disability' (RNID).

Registered Children's Nurse

A registered children's nurse (RCN) provides care across hospital and community, for those children with acute and chronic illness and those requiring palliative care. Inpatient care can vary in its complexity. Care is also provided in the patient's home and increasingly outreach and inreach integrated care programmes are being developed. The traditional segmentation of service from hospital to community is no longer appropriate for care of the child. An ambulatory care approach means more children can be cared for as close to home as possible, with only the sickest children having to be admitted to a tertiary centre where they can get the required care. In commenting on the educational programme that leads to the RCN qualification, An Bord Altranais states that:

> The children's/general nursing programme contains the essen-
> tial elements that facilitate the development of professional
> knowledge, skills and attitudes necessary to meet the nursing
> needs of clients along the lifespan continuum. Nursing the
> child with healthcare needs requires the adoption of a child
> and family centred philosophy within which each child and
> his/her family are valued. The aim of children's nursing is to
> facilitate child and family empowerment, and to enable main-
> tenance/restoration of optimal well being for the child in a
> needs-led culturally sensitive and high quality manner.[167]

Specialist hospitals for the care of sick infants and children have been
a feature of the health service in Ireland for close on two centuries.
The National Children's Hospital in Harcourt Street, Dublin, was
founded in 1821 and the Children's University Hospital, Temple
Street, Dublin, was founded in 1872. A third children's hospital,
Our Lady's Hospital for Sick Children in Crumlin, Dublin, was
founded in 1956.[168] The first school of paediatric nurse education
was established in the Temple Street Hospital in 1883. The *Nurses
Rules 2004*[169] replaced the title 'registered sick children's nurse' with
the title 'registered children's nurse' (RCN).

Public Health Nurse

Public health has been described as organised social and political
effort and health promotion for the benefit of populations, families and individuals.[170] There are over 2,400 public health nurses
(PHNs) on the active register, making them the largest group of
professionals working in the community.[171] PHNs practise as part
of a multidisciplinary team to deliver domiciliary care and have
a wide remit, encompassing primary, secondary and tertiary care
at three levels: individual, family and community.[172] They have
responsibility for providing a nursing service in the community to
multiple client groups with any type of condition, and public health
nursing is an amalgamation of services incorporating midwifery,
public health and home nursing.[173] Their role is threefold, combining that of manager, clinician and health promoter.[174]

The wide range of abilities and responsibilities of a PHN is
reflected in the educational and experiential preparation required
to register as one. Formerly, this took a minimum of eight years,

as the PHN until recently had to be registered as a general nurse and a registered midwife, had to have obtained a higher diploma in public health nursing and, in addition, have a minimum of two years' experience in clinical practice.[175] Under the *Nurses Rules 2004*,[176] nurses registered in divisions other than general nursing are eligible to apply for public health nursing courses, the requirement for a midwifery qualification has been removed and a module in maternity and child health has been substituted, reducing the preparation time to five years.[177]

Information on and analysis of the other divisions of the register (registered nurse tutor, registered nurse prescriber, advanced nurse practitioner and advanced midwife practitioner) is provided in Chapter 5 of this book, which deals with career pathways for nurses and midwives.

CHAPTER 4

Nursing and Midwifery Education

Nurse and Midwife Registration
Education Programmes

The recommendations in the *Report of the Commission on Nursing 1998*[178] resulted in a radical transformation of education programmes for nurses and midwives. Until then, general, psychiatric and intellectual disability (then known as mental handicap) nursing training was based on a three-year apprenticeship model. This system, irrespective of discipline, was based on classroom instruction and practical training, predominantly in a hospital setting. Student nurse training consisted of a student working on a ward and attending lectures. It was mainly characterised by a hospital-based training pattern where the student was an employee and part of the staffing complement of a hospital. The examination and assessment system consisted of continuous assessment of clinical skills through a proficiency assessment format and a final written examination conducted by An Bord Altranais.[179]

The apprenticeship model was evaluated by An Bord Altranais and a number of weaknesses were identified which militated against a beneficial experience for the student nurse. These included a lack of preparation for certain duties, a lack of clinical teaching, an emphasis on work rather than learning and an involvement in non-nursing duties. In the light of this evaluation, the traditional apprenticeship model of pre-registration nurse training and education was replaced by a new registration/diploma-based programme in general, psychiatric and mental handicap nursing. The diploma-based pre-registration education programme was offered by schools of nursing in association with colleges and universities. The objective of the transition to the new programme was to enhance nursing education and training and was in line with key recommendations contained in the report *The Future of Nurse Education and Training in Ireland*, published by An Bord Altranais in 1994.[180] The first nursing registration/diploma programme, following approval by An Bord Altranais, commenced on a pilot basis in University College Hospital, Galway, in association with the National University of Ireland, Galway (NUIG), in October 1994 and was rolled out throughout the rest of the country over the following four years.

The Commission on Nursing undertook an extensive consultation exercise on the programme during 1997 and 1998. While the introduction of the diploma programme was widely welcomed, there were concerns about its content and how it was being implemented. In addition, there were concerns relating to the very concept of the programme, which was seen by many as halfway between the traditional apprenticeship model of education and a degree programme, which did not offer nursing students the full educational and personal benefits of a third-level education. Students under the programme were not seen as 'real' third-level students and neither were they traditional apprentice students. The students had not been incorporated into the third-level student body. The schools of nursing under the registration/diploma programme still provided a substantial proportion of the theoretical and clinical education to student nurses. It was suggested that much of the education was still largely didactic and did not reflect the culture of self-directed learning in third-level education. It was also suggested that the programme did not reflect international trends in nursing education. Student nurses in Australia, New Zealand, Canada and the United States were being educated to degree level and in Northern Ireland the pre-registration education of student nurses had recently come under the aegis of Queen's University, Belfast.

In the literature review undertaken[181] on behalf of the Commission, the rationale for integrating pre-registration nursing education into the third-level sector at degree level was identified as the need to better prepare nurses for an ever more complex and technological system of healthcare provision.[182] There was a strong view that the nurse of the future required greater theoretical underpinning of the traditional clinical skills. Graduate education was viewed as offering nurses a more effective base on which to develop their practice skills and master a wide variety of skills. It was argued that the combination of sound formal education and reflective practice in a collegial atmosphere was most likely to produce expert practitioners.

In its final report, the Commission on Nursing recommended the following: the Minister for Health and Children should facilitate the transition of pre-registration nursing education into third-level institutes at degree level. Pre-registration nursing education in Ireland should be a third-level four-year honours degree programme. Transition to the degree programme should be nationwide and should start in the academic year 2002–2003. The programme should include theory and clinical practice in the three nursing divisions – general, psychiatric and mental handicap – and should include clinical placements, including twelve months' continuous placement as a paid employee of the health service. The academic year should be based around the existing academic calendars for third-level institutes and the Central Applications Office (CAO) should administer the application system for pre-registration education. A Nursing Education Forum[183] should be established to agree a strategy for the implementation of degree-level pre-registration education.

The Commission also recommended that a direct-entry midwifery course should be piloted in a midwifery hospital. This programme should initially be provided at diploma level but should also move to a degree programme in 2002. In relation to sick children's nursing, the Commission recommended that it should remain as a post-registration qualification.

In 2002, the full four-year honours pre-registration degree programme was introduced for general, psychiatric and mental handicap (later intellectual disability) nursing. For midwifery, in 2006, following a three-year direct-entry pilot programme, a four-year honours degree programme was introduced, leading to registration as a midwife. In children's nursing, the three-year children's nursing certificate course was discontinued in 1995 and from 1996 the only route to registration as a sick children's nurse was through an eighteen-month post-registration education programme. In 2006, an integrated children's and general nursing four-and-a-half-year undergraduate honours degree programme was introduced, leading to registration as a registered children's nurse and a registered general nurse.

In 2012, ten years after the introduction of the first pre-registration degree programme for nurses, the systems and structures for the delivery of these programmes are well established and entrenched within the academic institutions in Ireland. Nursing and midwifery has taken its place alongside all of the other healthcare disciplines within the academic system. Professors of nursing and midwifery, heads of school within the universities and institutes of technology, lecturers, senior lecturers and researchers are now an accepted part of the educational establishment. All of this is reflected in the requirements that are in place for the fulfilment of the standards required for registration of students as qualified nurses and midwives.

Overall, a minimum number of hours/weeks in theoretical and clinical instruction must be successfully completed before applying to register with An Bord Altranais. Table 2 summarises the requirements for each of the divisions of the register.[184]

Table 2: An Bord Altranais Requirements for Undergraduate Nursing and Midwifery Education Programmes

Programme	General, Intellectual Disability, Midwifery, Psychiatric	Children's and General Integrated
Theoretical instruction (to include self-directed study, exams)	58 weeks	70 weeks
Clinical instruction (supernumerary clinical placement)	40 weeks	54 weeks
Internship (inclusive of annual leave)	36 weeks	36 weeks
Other	10 weeks	10 weeks
Total minimum	**144 weeks**	**170 weeks**

For most of the programme, the student receives a combination of theoretical and clinical instruction and this period generally includes normal third-level college holidays. During this period, the student is not a paid employee of the health service. The usual entitlements and conditions regarding a means-tested third-level grant apply to student nurses.

The first clinical placement occurs early in the programme, usually within three months of commencement. A continual 36-week rostered clinical placement (internship) takes place during the fourth year. During this period, the student is a paid employee of the health service.

The National Qualifications Authority of Ireland (NQAI) has placed the nursing and midwifery undergraduate programmes at Level 8, honours bachelor degree, with Bachelor of Science (BSc) as the academic award. Five programmes are delivered at under-graduate degree level[185] (see Table 3).

Table 3: Programmes Leading to Registration with An Bord Altranais

Title	Duration	Leading to Registration
Children's and general nursing (integrated)	4.5 years	Registered children's nurse (RCN) and registered general nurse (RGN)
General nursing	4 years	Registered general nurse (RGN)
Intellectual disability nursing	4 years	Registered nurse intellectual disability (RNID)
Midwifery	4 years	Registered midwife (RM)
Psychiatric nursing	4 years	Registered psychiatric nurse (RPN)

Thirteen higher education institutes (HEIs) deliver 44 undergrad-uate degree programmes in partnership with 57 main healthcare agencies, providing 1,570 places in nursing and midwifery at pre-registration level[186] (see Table 4).

Table 4: Number of Programmes and Places

Programmes	Numbers and Places
Children's and general nursing (integrated)	4 programmes, with a total of 100 places, in 4 HEIs in association with 4 main healthcare agencies
General nursing	14 programmes, with a total of 860 places, in 13 HEIs in association with 22 main healthcare agencies
Intellectual disability nursing	8 programmes, with a total of 180 places, in 8 HEIs in association with 10 main healthcare agencies
Midwifery	6 programmes, with a total of 140 places, in 6 HEIs in association with 7 main healthcare agencies
Psychiatric nursing	12 programmes, with a total of 290 places, in 12 HEIs in association with 14 main healthcare agencies

Post-Registration Education

Nursing and Midwifery: A Career for You[187] contains information on a range of post-registration education programmes for nurses and midwives to acquire additional qualifications and qualify for entry to the register under more than one division of the register. An Bord Altranais operates a Nursing Career Centre,[188] where information and advice on these opportunities can be sourced.

There are five post-registration programmes leading to an additional registration with An Bord Altranais: children's nursing; midwifery; nurse tutor; public health nursing; and nurse prescriber. The programme in children's nursing is available at both pre-registration (i.e. integrated with general nursing as described above) and post-registration level. The midwifery programme is available at both pre-registration and post-registration levels.

Children's Nursing

For the post-registration children's nursing programme, a nurse who is registered in one of three divisions of the register – RNID, RPN and RGN – may apply to enter the post-registration RCN programme. The full-time programme is twelve months in duration. Successful completion of the programme entitles the applicant to apply for RCN registration and the award of a higher diploma from an HEI. The three HEIs and the three linked Dublin healthcare agencies offering the post-registration RCN programme are Dublin City University (DCU) and Children's University Hospital, Temple Street; Trinity College Dublin (TCD) and Adelaide and Meath Hospital incorporating the National Children's Hospital, Tallaght; and University College Dublin (UCD) and Our Lady's Children's Hospital, Crumlin.

Midwifery

The post-registration midwifery programme leading to the qualification of registered midwife is full-time and eighteen months in duration. An applicant must first be registered as a general nurse (RGN) before applying for the post-registration programme in midwifery. Successful completion of the programme entitles the applicant to apply for RM registration and the award of a higher diploma from a linked HEI. The seven maternity hospitals and linked HEIs currently offering the RM programme are Our Lady of Lourdes Hospital, Drogheda and Dundalk Institute of Technology (DkIT); University College Hospital, Galway and NUIG; the Coombe Women and Infants University Hospital and TCD; the Rotunda Hospital and TCD; Cork University Maternity Hospital and University College Cork (UCC); the National Maternity Hospital and UCD; and St Munchin's Regional Maternity Hospital and University of Limerick (UL).

Nurse Tutor

In order to qualify as a nurse tutor, a registered nurse or midwife must undertake a specific master's programme. On successful completion, the applicant is entitled to apply for registration as a nurse tutor (RNT). There is no separate register for midwife tutors. A nurse or midwife who is registered and who already holds a master's honours degree in nursing or midwifery or in an allied health science subject may, subject to the honours degree being deemed suitable by An Bord Altranais, undertake a further postgraduate qualification in education and subsequently apply for registration as a nurse tutor.

Public Health Nursing

In order to qualify for entry to the register as a public health nurse, an applicant must be registered as a general nurse (RGN). An RGN who is not registered as a midwife (RM) must also complete a child and maternal health module. Successful completion entitles the student to apply for PHN registration and an award from the HEI.

Nurse Prescriber

Registered nurses and midwives (RNID/RPN/RGN/RCN/RM) may also apply to undertake an education programme leading to registration as a nurse prescriber, which will equip them with the competencies to prescribe medications.[189] Education programmes leading to this qualification are run in cooperation with the schools of nursing in the Royal College of Surgeons in Ireland (RCSI), UCC, UCD and UL.

Registered general nurses and registered children's nurses may also apply to undertake an education programme in the prescribing of ionising radiation (X-rays). The education programmes must be approved by An Bord Altranais and successful completion will provide nurses with the authority to prescribe ionising radiation.[190]

Additional post-registration opportunities for nurses and midwives include opportunities to become a CNS/CMS and ANP/AMP. More detailed discussion on these opportunities can be found in Chapter 5 of this book, which deals with career pathways for nurses and midwives. In general, nurses and midwives who wish to become a CNS/CMS or ANP/AMP will require a postgraduate qualification. The minimum requirement for a CNS/CMS is a higher diploma (Level 8, NQAI) and for an ANP/AMP a master's (Level 9, NQAI). Candidates must also meet the criteria that have been defined by the National Council for these roles.[191] With the enactment of the Nurses and Midwives Act 2011 and the dissolution of the National Council, responsibility for this has now passed to An Bord Altranais and the HSE.

Maintaining Professional Competence

The Nurses and Midwives Act 2011[192] explicitly states that it is the duty of every registered nurse and midwife to maintain their professional competence and to be able to demonstrate that professional competence to the satisfaction of the Board. The Board is required to introduce a system or number of systems within one year of the commencement of this section of the Act designed to monitor the maintenance of professional competence by nurses and midwives. These are new provisions in the Act and represent a change from past practice. It is no longer optional for nurses and midwives to maintain their competence; they are required to do so by law and the law also requires the Board to put in place systems to ensure that this happens.

The maintenance of professional competence requires the adoption of a lifelong commitment to continuous professional development. This is an area to which the National Council had devoted considerable energy.

The National Council defined continuing professional development (CPD) as:

> [A] lifelong process, which includes both structured and informal activities that may include formal education programmes, participation in journal clubs, case conferencing, clinical

supervision, learning sets, preceptorship, mentorship, work-shops, distance learning programmes and reflection on practice. CPD encompasses processes, activities and experiences that contribute towards the development of a nurse or midwife, both personally and professionally.[193]

Further, the National Council adopted the definition of the related concept of lifelong learning as 'a continuously supportive process which stimulates and empowers individuals to acquire all the knowledge, values, skills and understanding they will require throughout their lifetimes, and to apply them with competence, creativity, and enjoyment in all roles, circumstances and environments'.[194]

The National Council referred to what are called the components and attributes of competence resulting in effective and/or superior performance. These include practical and technical skills, communication and interpersonal skills, organisational and managerial skills, the ability to practise safely and effectively, utilising evidence-based practice, having a problem-solving approach to care, utilising critical thinking, being part of the multidisciplinary team, demonstrating a professional attitude, accepting responsibility and being accountable for one's practice.

One of the factors impeding participation in CPD by all nurses and midwives is access. Nurses and midwives living and working in more remote areas of the country may find it difficult to get time off to attend educational courses and activities that are held in centres far from their place of work. One possible solution is electronic learning or e-learning: web-based initiatives designed to provide access to CPD opportunities. The 'eLearning Guru'[195] provided by the HSE performance and development website describes a wide range of advantages inherent in this approach. The Nurses and Midwives Act 2011 includes a determination that employers have a duty to facilitate the maintenance of professional competence by nurses and midwives, including the provision of learning opportunities in the workplace.[196]

The importance of CPD in the lives of nurses and midwives was one of the motivating factors behind the publication by the National Council of guidelines on portfolio development for nurses and midwives.[197] The guidelines were aimed at individual nurses and midwives working at the forefront of healthcare delivery, to assist them to identify, reflect upon and record the contribution they make to direct and indirect care, encourage them to store records of their development in a coherent and structured manner and provide guidance and information on achieving their individual professional goals within the context of the needs of the health service. These guidelines were published at a time when there was no legal or statutory requirement for nurses and midwives to engage in CPD. The popularity of the publications[198] was quoted by the National Council as evidence that nurses and midwives were very willing to engage in CPD. The provisions of the new Act in this regard will make the use of portfolio development even more relevant.

The National Council published three reports on the future professional development of nursing and midwifery.

- *Agenda for the Future Professional Development of Nursing and Midwifery.*[199] The National Council conducted a nationwide consultation from March 2002 to March 2003. Workshops were held with directors of nursing and midwifery, directors of the nursing and midwifery planning and development units (NMPDUs), and nurses and midwives from all divisions of the register. A call for submissions yielded 105 written responses. The report benchmarked progress to date for general, mental health, children's, intellectual disability and older person nursing and midwifery and set the agenda for a debate on options, direction and actions for the future. CPD emerged as the predominant issue in this report for all areas of nursing and was viewed as vital to developing nursing and midwifery practice in modern health structures.
- *Report on the Continuing Professional Development of Staff Nurses and Staff Midwives.*[200] This report reviewed the CPD activities of staff nurses and midwives, competency achievement and maintenance relevant to service need and personal professional development, and the career choice relevant to CPD and competency of staff nurses and staff midwives. The data collection methods for this report included a literature review, focus groups and questionnaire. Staff nurses from general, mental health, intellectual disability and children's nursing and midwives were invited to participate. Nurses and midwives from cities, towns and rural areas were represented, as were those working in community and inpatient settings. Recommendations covered the development of structures

to support CPD for staff nurses and midwives. The report contained a detailed table of recommendations that summarised the objectives, the deliverables and the responsibilities of individual stakeholders in this area.

- *Agenda for the Future Professional Development of Public Health Nursing.*[201] A nationwide consultation was carried out from November 2004 to February 2005. Workshops were held with directors of public health nursing, assistant directors of public health nursing, public health nurses engaged in clinical practice and other key stakeholders. The main concerns expressed by participants related to role clarity, workload demands, variation in service provision and delivery of care, the clinical career pathway, leadership, skill mix and multidisciplinary teamworking. The report benchmarked progress on professional development to date and set an agenda for future actions.

The Future of Nursing and Midwifery Education

The introduction of degree-based pre-registration education for nurses and midwives in Ireland has raised a number of issues that require further discussion. One such issue is the advisability of moving towards a common point of entry for the professions versus the maintenance of the current system based on five different points of entry, and an assessment of the implications of the Bologna Declaration[202] (the joint declaration by the European Ministers of Education; see Appendix 1) for pre-registration nursing and midwifery education in Ireland.

The introduction of a common point-of-entry system for nursing and midwifery in Ireland would be in line with existing systems in the UK and most other countries with a degree programme for preregistration nurse education. The common point of entry would entail all nurse and midwife students sharing a common first year or eighteen months at university and then choosing to specialise in a particular branch. The advantages of such a system would be the creation of greater intradisciplinary solidarity within the professions and the development of common standards across all the branches of the professions. As it stands, Ireland is the only country that has five separate degree programmes (general, children's, psychiatric and intellectual disability nursing and midwifery). This is not likely to be sustainable in the future.

In June 2004, An Bord Altranais commissioned what became known as the Five Points Project[203] to examine the rationale for and impact of maintaining the five points of entry. The study concluded with a series of recommendations that summarised the overall approach to pre-registration entry to nursing and midwifery education prevailing in Ireland today, where there is a four-year degree programme with a 36-week internship clinical placement in the fourth year.[204]

In 2011, the Department of Health commenced a review of the undergraduate nursing and midwifery degree programmes in order to assess their efficiency and effectiveness in preparing nurses and midwives to practise in the Irish healthcare system, now and into the future. The review is guided by a review group representing key stakeholders. Terms of reference for the Strategic Review of the Undergraduate Nursing and Midwifery Degree Programmes state that 'The review group has been established to oversee a review of the nursing and midwifery programmes having regard to the objectives of the current health reform programme, the future workforce needs of the public health system and the need to achieve value for money.'[205]

The review is being conducted on a modular basis, consisting of two elements. First, it will consist of an examination of the content of the undergraduate programmes and of the structure of the current degree programmes, including the separate points of entry, clinical placement requirements and governance requirements. Second, it will provide an analysis of the number of student places required to ensure that there are sufficient numbers of nurse and midwife graduates for new patterns of service delivery within the public health system. Following the completion of both of these exercises, the Department of Education and Skills and the Higher Education Authority (HEA), in consultation with the HEIs, will lead on the development of any changes required in relation to the organisation and delivery of nursing and midwifery degree programmes within the higher education system. This will take into account the broader education policy considerations in relation to demand for such programmes nationally and internationally and the overall funding implications involved. It will also take into account full consideration of the findings of the report to the Minister for Health on workforce planning and curricula changes.

In March 2012, the Department of Health published a report on the results of a consultation exercise carried out by the review group.[206] A total of 225 written submissions were received, 18 focus groups were held covering nursing, midwifery and public interest and an additional 22 stakeholder groups meetings were held. There was strong support for the degree programme in the consultation process. Suggestions were made to improve programme oversight, delivery and evaluation. Consideration should be given to a standard curriculum, assessment process and documentation. An Bord Altranais should provide greater guidance and changes were suggested to the requirements and standards for nurse and midwife education programmes published by An Bord Altranais. General support for the five points of entry remained; however, the concepts of shared learning, common foundation subjects and interdisciplinary education were advocated. Learning outcomes and specific competencies for each year of the programmes were seen to be essential. A philosophy of patient empowerment, population health improvement and lifelong learning were advocated. A principles-based approach to the curriculum driven by emerging models of healthcare delivery in Ireland was advocated which would support national consistency where graduates attain specific competencies at the end of their programmes of education.

Any review of pre-registration nursing and midwifery education, however, would also necessarily have to look in detail at the benefits and opportunities presented by the possibility of a common point of entry and interdisciplinary education. The context and environment in which nursing and midwifery graduates are prepared to practise is evolving and is common to all divisions of the register. It is interesting to note that one of the outcomes of the consultation exercise was general support for the five points of entry while at the same time recognising the need for more shared learning, common foundation subjects and interdisciplinary education. The question of duplication of infrastructure and of funding for higher education programmes was highlighted by the HEA in its publication *Towards a Future Higher Education Landscape*.[207] It is probably unavoidable that this question will be addressed in the context of the overall reform of higher education.

While it is timely that a detailed review of the degree programme should be conducted now, almost six years after the first cohort of students have completed their degrees and qualified to register as nurses and midwives, there is an important dimension that is missing from this review. In addition to the question of content of the curriculum, workforce planning and value for money, consideration should also be given to the impact of educational attainment on clinical outcomes. This is not included in the terms of reference of the review. Consideration should be given to a separate study that looks at this.

A review of the impact of educational attainment on clinical outcomes would require the collection and analysis of data on issues such as patient satisfaction, quality of care, clinical outcomes and other criteria. Such an analysis should be conducted in the context of changes in the delivery of healthcare and the ongoing reform of the processes and structures within the system. It would provide valuable information to inform programme delivery, taking into account current and future service needs.

An example of a relevant quantitative study[208] on the effects of levels of nursing education on patient outcomes can be found in the United States, which set out to determine whether the educational levels of registered nurses in hospitals had a measurable effect on patient outcomes. It found that a 10 per cent increase in the proportion of nurses holding a bachelor's degree was associated with a 5 per cent decrease in both the likelihood of patients dying within 30 days of admission and the odds of failure to rescue. The conclusion of the study was that, in hospitals with higher proportions of nurses educated at the baccalaureate level or higher, surgical patients experienced lower mortality and failure to rescue rates.

The National Council also commissioned extensive research on the impact of educational attainment and specialisation in nursing and midwifery in clinical settings.[209] This research provided strong evidence that these developments in nursing and midwifery education and training have had a significant impact in clinical settings. This will be discussed in more detail in Chapter 5 of this book, which will look at the various career pathways open to nurses and midwives as a result of the developments that have taken place since the publication of the *Report of the Commission on Nursing*.

An Bord Altranais is responsible for defining the standards and requirements for nurse and midwife education programmes. There are many changes taking place within the health services as part of the ongoing health reform programme. These changes have significant implications for the roles of nurses and midwives and it is important that the educational programmes are designed in a manner that takes account of these changes and equip nurses and midwives with the knowledge and skills they require to adapt. It is important, therefore, that timely reviews of the standards and requirements for nurse and midwife education requirements are carried out by An Bord Altranais. It is interesting to note that this also emerged as one of the conclusions of the consultation report produced by the review group.

International Trends in Nursing and Midwifery Education

The Bologna Declaration

Membership of the European Union is a key influence on how Ireland delivers its education for nurses and midwives. Of particular relevance in this regard is what is known as the Bologna Declaration.[210] This was a joint declaration by Ministers of Education from the member states of the European Union that set out to create a coherent, compatible and competitive European Higher Education Area by 2010 (see Appendix 1).

The main objectives of the Bologna Declaration include creation of comparable, uniform and easily readable degrees through a European Credit Transfer System, promotion of EU-wide quality assurance based on comparable criteria and methodologies, and promotion of lifelong learning and removal of obstacles to mobility in the EU.[211]

Although the European Commission was not an initiator of the Bologna process, it had an increasingly important role in helping to achieve its aims and objectives. European Union Directive 2005/36/EC was transposed into Irish law in 2008 and repealed previous directives. It has implications for recognition of qualifications of nurses and midwives educated and trained in other member states who wish to travel and work as registered nurses or midwives in Ireland.[212] The European Commission published a Green Paper, *Modernising the Professional Qualifications Directive (Directive 2005/36/EC)*,[213] which includes arrangements for recognition of nursing, midwifery and other health professional qualifications across Europe and common minimum standards for nurse and midwife education. The Green Paper was aimed at gathering stakeholders' views on modernisation of the Directive. Over 400 submissions were received and results of the consultation and general updates were provided by the end of 2011.

In October 2010 the HEA and NQAI in Ireland published a review they had commissioned on Ireland's participation in the

Bologna process entitled *Taking Stock: Ten Years of the Bologna Process in Ireland*.[214] The review noted that the European Higher Education Area (EHEA) had been launched in 2010 and, by March 2010, the cohort of participating countries had grown from 29 to 47. The review reports that the undergraduate/postgraduate degree structure proposed in the Declaration has been modified into a three-cycle system, which now incorporates the concept of qualifications frameworks, with an emphasis on learning outcomes. The countries that have signed the Bologna Declaration have agreed to implement student-centred, outcome-based and transparent higher educational programmes on the basis of three sequential cycles: the bachelor, the master and the doctorate.

The Tuning Educational Structures in Europe Programme is an initiative by a number of universities throughout Europe interested in taking up the Bologna challenge.[215] They approached the European Commission for financial assistance in the framework of the Socrates programme[216] and through the European Universities Association they widened the group of participants. Phase 1 of the programme focused on identifying points of reference for generic and subject-specific competencies of first- and second-cycle graduates in a series of subject areas (business administration, education sciences, geology, history, mathematics, physics and chemistry). Nursing was added to the list of subject areas in phase 2. The programme is coordinated by the University of Deusto in Spain and the University of Groningen in The Netherlands. The name 'Tuning' was adopted to indicate that the universities involved were not seeking total harmonisation of their degree programmes nor a unified, prescriptive, definitive European curriculum, but rather they were looking for points of reference, convergence and common understanding. The programme aims to protect the rich diversity of European education and is not intended to restrict the independence of academic and subject specialisation or to damage the local and national academic authority.[217]

One of the aims of the Tuning Project is the development of a transparent common language in the description of higher education programmes in order to enhance comparability and to foster their international recognition.[218] A guide to defining key programme competencies and writing good degree programme learning outcomes is provided. Nursing is identified as a good example of this (see Table 5).

Table 5: Sample Learning Outcomes – Nursing

Level	Programme Learning Outcome
First cycle/Bachelor's	The nurse can work closely with individuals, groups and carers, using a range of skills to carry out comprehensive, systematic and holistic assessments. The assessments must take into account current and previous physical, social, cultural, psychological, spiritual, genetic and environmental factors that may be relevant to individuals and their families.
Second cycle/Master's	In his/her designated speciality, the nurse must demonstrate his/her mastery of advanced nursing skills (including diagnostic and therapeutic techniques) to assess and manage patients with complex health/illness states.
Clinical Doctorate	The nurse can demonstrate leadership in his/her chosen clinical area, and is able to influence and set strategic practice development and research agendas.
Doctorate/PhD	The nurse can demonstrate a systematic acquisition and understanding of a substantial body of knowledge which is at the forefront of the discipline of nursing, or an area of professional nursing practice.

The educational system is now underpinned by European standards and guidelines for quality assurance. The most visible element of the Bologna process, from the perspective of the higher education community generally, is the suite of 'instruments' developed to address the objectives of the Declaration.[219] Of particular note is the infrastructure of qualifications frameworks now under construction throughout European higher education. This comprises national frameworks of higher education qualifications, to be introduced in all participating countries, and a European 'meta-framework' to which national systems can relate, the Framework of Qualifications for the European Higher Education Area (FQEHEA). Ireland has already produced its own National Framework of Qualifications (NFQ) and the HEA/NQAI review[220] notes that this, together with the European Qualifications Framework (EQF), will greatly facilitate the worldwide recognition of Irish qualifications. This, according to the review, provides Ireland with an opportunity to become internationally recognised and ranked as a world leader in the delivery of high-quality international education.

The World Health Organisation

In 2005 the World Health Organisation (WHO) regional office for Europe undertook a review of basic nursing and midwifery education programmes in Europe.[221] The review noted that, while there was a general move across Europe to university-based education at diploma or degree level for nurses and midwives, there were wide discrepancies on issues such as age at entry level, qualifications and content of the curriculum.

The WHO has clearly signalled its support for a move towards degree-level education in a number of reports and strategy documents, including *Nurses and Midwives for Health: WHO European Strategy for Nursing and Midwifery Education*,[222] which identified a baccalaureate degree as a prerequisite for professional practice. This has also been supported by the Nursing and Midwifery Council (NMC) in the UK and by the review of education that has been conducted in Australia.[223]

In 2009, the WHO published *Global Standards for the Initial Education of Professional Nurses and Midwives*.[224] These 'global standards' were intended to serve as a benchmark in moving towards a common competency-based outcome of education and learning systems. This is particularly important in an age of increasing globalisation, where the greater part of the global healthcare workforce consists of an estimated 35 million nurses and midwives.[225]

The kick-start to the development of the standards was provided by a meeting of key stakeholders convened in May 2005 by the WHO. The purpose of the meeting was to examine the contribution of nursing and midwifery to the millennium goals. The standards were subsequently developed over the next three years, under the guidance and oversight of a planning group led by the WHO and Sigma Theta Tau International.

The goal of the global standards is to establish educational criteria and assure outcomes that are based on evidence and competency, that promote the progressive nature of education and lifelong learning and that ensure the employment of practitioners who are competent and who, by providing quality care, promote positive health outcomes in the populations they serve. This has resulted in standards relating to outcomes, governance, accreditation, faculty and programme admission.

The standards state that graduates should demonstrate established competencies in nursing and midwifery practice and a sound understanding of the determinants of health. They also state that graduates of an initial programme in nursing or midwifery must meet regulatory body standards, leading to professional licensure/registration as a nurse or a midwife. Graduates should also be awarded a professional degree and should be eligible for entry into advanced education programmes.

The standards also state that nursing or midwifery schools should employ methods to track the professional success and progression of education of each graduate and graduates will be knowledge-able practitioners who adhere to the code of ethics and standards of the profession. The schools of nursing or midwifery should prepare graduates who demonstrate use of evidence in practice, cultural competence, the ability to practise in the healthcare systems of their respective countries and meet population needs, critical and analytical thinking, the ability to manage resources and practise safely and effectively, the ability to be effective client advocates and professional partners with other disciplines in healthcare delivery, community service orientation, leadership ability and continual professional development.

CHAPTER 5

Career Pathways in Nursing and Midwifery

The Commission on Nursing

The *Report of the Commission on Nursing*, published in 1998, represented the most comprehensive review of nursing and midwifery ever conducted in Ireland. The Commission was established following a period of considerable industrial unrest among nurses and midwives about the conditions under which they were employed, the career development options open to them, the nature and range of educational services available and the general perception of the professions. In 1997, nurses and midwives voted for strike action. The setting up of the Commission on Nursing by the Government, following a recommendation from the Labour Court, averted a strike.[226]

The agreed terms of reference for the work of the Commission were that it should examine and report on the role of nurses in the health services, including the evolving role of nurses, reflecting their professional development and their role in the overall management of services; promotional opportunities and related difficulties; structural and work changes appropriate for the effective and efficient discharge of that role; the requirements placed on nurses, both in training and the delivery of services; segmentation of the grade; and training and educational requirements.[227]

The original terms of reference also stated that, in its recommendations, the Commission should seek 'to provide a secure basis for the further development of nursing in the context of anticipated changes in health services, their organisation and delivery'. In light of discussions during the Commission's consultation process, and following agreement by An Bord Altranais, the Commission sought and secured an extension of its terms of reference to include 'the role and function of An Bord Altranais generally, including, inter alia, education and professional development, regulation and protection of the citizen'.

One of the recommendations of the Commission on Nursing was that a monitoring committee would be established that would issue yearly reports on the implementation of its recommendations (this committee was established and held its first meeting on 1 February 2000). It was envisaged that recommendations without a suggested timescale would be implemented as soon as practicable and, in any event, by the end of 2002. The Commission, in addition to timescales given in its report, identified four recommendations as urgent: the establishment of the Nursing Education Forum (for pre-registration education); the establishment of the National Council (for post-registration education); the establishment of the NMPDUs in each health board, all of which should be established at the earliest possible date; and the introduction of legislation amending the Nurses Act 1985,[228] which should be introduced before the Oireachtas by early 1999. Three of the four were implemented within a year or two of the publication of the report. The fourth, involving the amending of the legislation, was not implemented until 2011.

The Commission's report provided a comprehensive framework, or blueprint, for the development of the professions into the future. This included the creation of a number of new bodies with responsibility for the development of the professions, such as the nursing policy division in the Department of Health and Children, the NMPDUs and the National Council.

Two of the most far-reaching recommendations of the report were the introduction of a pre-registration degree programme for nurses and midwives superseding/succeeding the certificate and diploma programmes as the qualifying programme for entry to the professions, and the determination of a comprehensive clinical career pathway, from generalist nurse to CNS to ANP. An equivalent career pathway was introduced for midwives, from generalist midwife to CMS to AMP. The report introduced for the first time in Ireland the concept of CNS/CMS and ANP/AMP as part of the clinical career pathway for nurses and midwives. The implementation of these recommendations has transformed the professions in recent years and promises to provide a platform for the further development of the contribution of the professions to the health services of the future.

Development of the Clinical Career Pathway

Until 1998, there was no framework for developing a clinical career pathway in Ireland, although there were some initiatives at a local level aimed at developing specialists in nursing. Thus, for example, in 1996, the first nurse acknowledged to be practising at an advanced level in Ireland was appointed on a pilot basis in an emergency department in a Dublin hospital and was known as an emergency nurse practitioner. Also in 1996, the *Tender for the Establishment and Provision of Cardiac Surgery Services at St James's Hospital* in Dublin contained a proposal to include four nurse practitioner posts as part of the staffing complement.[229]

The roots of specialisation in nursing and midwifery in Ireland can be found in the *Report of the Working Party on General Nursing*,[230] published in 1980, which recommended the appointment of specialist nurses to enhance nursing care by providing specialist nursing advice to other nurses. It was the *Report of the Commission on Nursing* that recommended the establishment of a comprehensive clinical career pathway framework to encourage experienced nurses and midwives to remain in clinical practice and use their expert skills to improve patient outcomes and respond to health policy developments. The clinical career pathway leads from generalist to specialist to advanced practice. Levels on the pathway are linked with levels of educational preparation, responsibility and autonomy, and to different points on a pay scale that reflect these different levels of responsibility. Responsibility for monitoring the development of the clinical career pathway framework was assigned to the National Council.

The clinical career pathway is designed to ensure that nurses and midwives could fulfil their professional role within a range of care settings and working at different grades and with different levels of clinical autonomy. These grades include those of the generalist nurse at staff nurse and staff midwife grade, the specialist nurse/midwife at CNS/CMS grade and the advanced practice nurse/midwife at ANP/AMP grade.[231] The respective roles of staff nurses, staff midwives, CNSs, CMSs, ANPs and

AMPs are distinguished by their scope of practice, educational preparation and levels of clinical decision-making, responsibility and autonomy.

One of the provisions contained in the Nurses and Midwives Act 2011 was the dissolution of the National Council, which had been established as an independent statutory agency[232] with responsibility for the development of a clinical career pathway for nurses and midwives. It was responsible for determining the appropriate level of qualification and experience necessary for entry into specialist practice and advanced practice for nursing and midwifery. In addition, the National Council provided a range of professional development and support services appropriate to each step on the clinical career pathway. These included the provision of funding to support additional continuing educational initiatives for nurses and midwives in cooperation with the NMPDUs. The National Council also worked closely with the NMPDUs on a wide range of strategic development issues, which included the development of clinical specialist and advanced practitioner posts and the promotion of research in nursing and midwifery.

The National Council took the lead in the introduction of important policy initiatives, such as the involvement of nurses and midwives in prescribing medicinal preparations (in partnership with An Bord Altranais), the promotion of research in nursing and midwifery (in partnership with the Health Research Board) and the promotion of educational programmes to support the clinical career pathway (in partnership with third-level institutions and the centres of nurse and midwife education). The National Council also provided master classes and seminars on nursing and midwifery topics, organised an annual conference on professional development issues and provided an interactive portal website that acted as host for a wide range of nursing and midwifery specialist interest groups. The National Council also offered extensive professional advice at individual and organisational levels.

The National Council was a leader in the strategic development of roles within the health services. It was unique in that it worked with both the public and the private sectors. Thus, for example, ANP/AMP and CNS/CMS posts have been established in many public and private/voluntary institutions throughout Ireland. To do this, the National Council developed frameworks that defined the roles of the CNS/CMS and the ANP/AMP. It also set out the core concepts of these roles and provided guidance on how they should be established.[233] The National Council also required ANPs/AMPs to apply for re-accreditation after five years. This kind of strategic role development was a new concept in international terms and had been adopted in only a few countries, such as Australia, New Zealand and Ireland, mainly as a result of lessons learned from countries such as Canada and the UK, where a lack of role definition as well as clarity of nomenclature, scope of practice and education level had caused considerable confusion among both the nursing profession and the general public.[234]

Some of the functions of the National Council had already transferred to An Bord Altranais under the provisions of SI No 3 of 2010 – Health (An Bord Altranais) (Additional Functions) Order 2010.[235] Under the terms of this statutory instrument (SI), An Bord Altranais was required to create a division of the register for ANPs/AMPs and to determine, in accordance with criteria set by the National Council, applications for the accreditation of posts and of individuals as ANPs/AMPs. An Bord Altranais was also required to monitor the register to ensure that individuals were removed from the register if they no longer complied with the criteria set by the National Council or if their employment in the post as ANP/AMP had ceased. This SI had the effect of providing strong protection for the title of ANP/AMP and of linking the role to a specific post. In other words, it was not possible to use the title ANP/AMP unless one was actually employed in a role that had been accredited and approved by the Board. These requirements were formalised in a new edition of the *Nurses Rules 2010*.[236] Rules 5.11 and 5.12 made provision for the admission to the register of those candidates who met the criteria set by the National Council for the roles of ANP and AMP respectively. Rules 8.1 to 8.4 made provision for the accreditation of ANP/AMP posts and for the removal of accreditation from any ANP/AMP who no longer met the criteria set by the National Council.

Following the enactment of the provisions of SI No 3 of 2010, all paper and electronic files held by the National Council in relation to advanced nurse/midwife practitioner posts and post-holders were transferred to An Bord Altranais.

The development of specialist practice at the level of CNS/CMS was not covered by the SI and the National Council continued to set the criteria and standards for these roles. Service providers within the health services could make an application to the National Council for a determination that a particular post and a specific individual met the criteria. Once a determination had been made by the National Council, a qualified person who met the criteria could be appointed as a CNS/CMS. In accordance with its statutory function, the National Council continued to monitor CNS/CMS posts at a national level in partnership with the eight NMPDUs. By 15 November 2011, 2,333 CNS/CMS posts had either been approved or been deemed to have met the National Council's standards and criteria for approval.

The Nurses and Midwives Act 2011 repealed SI No 3 of 2010. However, pending the introduction of the commencement orders for the implementation of the Act, it will continue to be in force. Once the Act has been fully implemented, it will be the responsibility of the Board to set the criteria and standards that should apply to the development of specialisation within nursing and midwifery at both ANP/AMP and CNS/CMS levels and to make determinations in relation to applications from service providers in relation to compliance. ANPs/AMPs will also be included on the register maintained by the Board. This will not be a requirement for CNSs/CMSs, although it is expected that the Board will monitor these posts and develop a system for tracking those nurses and midwives who have been deemed as meeting the standard and criteria set for these posts.

In December 2011, all paper and electronic files held by the National Council in relation to CNS/CMS posts and post-holders were transferred to An Bord Altranais in line with the Data Protection Acts of 1988 and 2003[237] and An Bord Altranais became the data controller in relation to these files. All CNSs/CMSs and directors of nursing and midwifery were informed of the file transfer.

The impetus for the future development of specialisation in nursing and midwifery at both ANP/AMP and CNS/CMS levels will now need to come from the services. The Nurses and Midwives Act 2011 (part 10, section 84) explicitly states that it is the responsibility of the HSE to promote the development of specialist nursing and midwifery education and training and to coordinate such development in cooperation with the Board and the nursing and midwifery training bodies approved by the Board. The HSE is also required, in cooperation with the nursing and midwifery training bodies and after consultation with the HEA, to undertake appropriate nursing and midwifery workforce planning for the purpose of meeting specialist nursing and midwifery staffing and training needs of the public health services on an ongoing basis. The

HSE is also responsible for advising the Minister in relation to these matters.

The future development of specialisation in nursing and midwifery at CNS/CMS and ANP/AMP levels is dependent, therefore, on the leadership and initiative of the HSE and the support and cooperation of the Board and the educational institutions. It should be noted, however, that the Nurses and Midwives Act 2011 confers certain responsibilities on the HSE in relation to the development of specialisation in public health services. The National Council did not confine its activities only to public health services. It worked with nursing and midwife professionals in both the public and the private/voluntary services. The Board is perhaps the only body that can provide the necessary leadership across the whole of the professions and its role in promoting awareness of the criteria and guidelines for the development of these roles will be a very important part of ensuring that developments span public and private service provision.

Current Career Pathways

The first step in the career pathway for nurses and midwives is the pre-registration undergraduate degree programme that equips them with the knowledge, skills and competencies necessary to enable them to have their name entered on the register maintained by An Bord Altranais. Of course, it is important to point out that there are many nurses and midwives in the health services who qualified before the introduction of the degree programme, having come through the apprenticeship model or the diploma model. They carry with them the expertise they have gained over the years of their service and qualify for participation in all steps of the career pathway. For all nurses and midwives, progress along the career pathway is made possible by additional and ongoing continuing professional development and the acquisition of further competencies.

This journey is often referred to in the terms originally coined by Patricia Benner[238] as a journey from novice to expert. Benner applies the Dreyfuss[239] model of skill acquisition to nursing. She states that a nurse will pass through five levels of proficiency: novice, advanced beginner, competent, proficient and expert. The novice stage includes the pre-registration education and clinical practice period leading up to acceptance on the register. The advanced beginner phase is considered to last for a period of eighteen months post-registration, during which the nurse or midwife is gaining experience and learning how to apply the knowledge and skills that have been learned in the novice stage. To become competent, Benner estimates that it takes between eighteen months and three years of practice in the same area, learning how to make sense of the situation and to apply rules and plan care. During this phase, the nurse/midwife learns how to apply a systematic approach to care. During this period, the nurse or midwife may also undertake further postgraduate study in an area of clinical practice at higher diploma level. To arrive at the level of proficient and expert, Benner estimates that it will take a minimum of three years for the former and five years for the latter. The timeline will vary for each individual and will be in direct proportion to how much the nurse or midwife has invested in his/her own development and acquisition of critical thinking skills over the years.

There are three broad career pathways open to nurses and midwives: clinical, management, and education and research.

Clinical Career Pathway

Once a nurse or midwife has completed his or her pre-registration education, the entry level on the clinical career pathway is as a staff nurse/staff midwife on the register. Staff nurses and staff midwives are integral members of the multidisciplinary team providing significant clinical care for individuals and families in a wide range of settings, including acute, community, residential and extended care settings and homes. They provide comprehensive patient assessments to develop, implement and evaluate an integrated plan of healthcare, and provide evidence-based nursing and midwifery interventions. The staff nurse or midwife engages in monitoring and evaluating the patient's response to interventions and treatment.

Progression along the clinical career pathway may include the acquisition of additional academic knowledge and clinical skills in a specialised area such as to enable them to become recognised as a CNS or CMS. CNSs/CMSs work with the multidisciplinary team to provide specialised assessment, planning, delivery and evaluation of care using protocol-driven guidelines. Care delivery and caseload management is delivered in line with core concepts (clinical focus, patient/client advocacy, education and training, audit and research, and consultancy).[240]

An additional role on the clinical career pathway is that of ANP or AMP. The caseload of ANPs/AMPs involves holistic assessment, diagnosis, autonomous decision-making regarding treatment, provision of interventions and discharge from a full episode of care. ANPs and AMPs provide care delivery and caseload management in line with core concepts (autonomy in clinical practice, expert practice, professional and clinical leadership, and research).[241]

The National Council defined the criteria and competencies for recognition at each stage along the career pathway in the form of a framework for the establishment of posts at clinical specialist and advanced practice levels.[242] In order to be able to use the title CNS/ CMS or ANP/AMP, a nurse or midwife must demonstrate that they have attained the required level of academic qualifications and that they meet the criteria defined by the National Council for these posts. Once the Nurses and Midwives Act 2011 becomes operational, the criteria for these posts will be set and monitored by the Nursing and Midwifery Board of Ireland.

In addition, the National Council published a number of position papers on the development of specialist and advanced practitioner roles in emergency departments,[243] intellectual disability services,[244] older persons nursing,[245] and midwifery.[246] These position papers provide detailed guidance on the assessment of service need and on the approach to be adopted in determining the need. The guidance provided on service needs analysis augments that already provided in the National Council publication *Service Needs Analysis for Clinical Nurse/Midwife Specialists and Advanced Nurse/Midwife Practitioners*,[247] which provides advice and a template for the preparation of a business case to support the development of new roles.

Management Career Pathway

On the management career pathway, the top grade is the role of director of nursing or director of midwifery, which is an executive corporate role within a hospital or institutional setting, and the director of public health nursing, responsible for the nursing and midwifery resource that operates within the community setting. The middle grade is made up of assistant directors of nursing/ midwifery in both hospital and community settings. They take responsibility for the operational and professional management of divisions within institutions or community healthcare settings. They are usually supported in this role by clinical nurse/midwife managers (CNMs/CMMs), a central position in the operational management of front-line care. The CNM/CMM is usually responsible for the management of a unit or ward within the institution.

There are three CNM/CMM grades. CNM1/CMM1 is at assistant ward sister level and frequently deputises for the CNM2/ CMM2. The CNM3/CMM3 is used in institutional settings where there are a number of wards or units within a division, with a number of CNM2/CMM2 grade managers who require coordination. This might occur, for example, in a large acute care hospital where there are many operating theatres, each run by a CNM2/ CMM2. The overall coordination of the nursing resource within the theatre services would then be the responsibility of the CNM3/ CMM3. Similar considerations would apply to other divisions within the hospital.

The Commission on Nursing highlighted the importance of the role of management in nursing and midwifery and, as a result of its recommendations, much work has been done in recent years on identifying the key competencies that are required of nurse and midwife managers. The Office for Health Management (OHM) (whose functions have now been integrated into the HSE's performance and development unit) has been instrumental in the past in healthcare leadership and management training for professional and non-professional groups within the health service, including nurses and midwives. Specific initiatives included the preparation of personal development plans, a nursing competency framework, a mentoring programme and the CIM initiative.

In December 2004 the OHM published a directory of competency development options, which was intended to complement the existing competency-related tools and initiatives for managers in all disciplines within the health services. This included a management competency user pack for nurse and midwife managers,[248] to assist employers and managers in raising understanding of the competencies required at this level and to give practical guidance on how these competencies could be developed and enhanced. The OHM identified a number of core competencies that should be present in managers at different levels within the health services. These are listed in Table 6.

Table 6: Nurse and Midwife Management Competencies[249]

Generic nursing and midwifery management competencies	1. Promotion of evidence-based decision-making 2. Building and maintaining relationships 3. Communication and influencing skills 4. Service initiation and innovation 5. Resilience and composure 6. Integrity and ethical stance 7. Sustained personal commitment 8. Practitioner competence and professional credibility
Additional Competencies	
Front-line nursing management level	Leading on clinical practice and service quality Planning and organisation of activities and resources Building and leading a team
Mid-level nursing management	Empowering and enabling leadership style Proactive approach to planning Effective coordination of resources Setting and monitoring performance standards Negotiation skills
Top-level nursing management	Leading on vision, values and processes Strategic and systems thinking Working at corporate level Establishing policy, systems and structures Developmental approach to staff

Education Career Pathway

Since the introduction of the pre-registration nursing and midwifery degree programmes in 2002, many rich opportunities have emerged for nurses and midwives in the area of education and research. Universities and other third-level institutions have created faculties, schools or departments of nursing and midwifery with a career structure that includes progression from lecturer to senior lecturer or professor within the institution. In addition, large hospitals with centres for nurse or midwifery education (CNE/CME) also offer educational career development opportunities, including roles as clinical placement coordinators, practice development coordinators, tutors and directors of the centres.

Research

Research has become an important part of the development of the professions. The requirement for evidence-based practice is integral to the delivery of safe patient-centred healthcare. Clinical research facilities for nursing and midwifery have emerged in response to the recommendation of the Commission on Nursing that nurses and midwives should be involved in medical-led clinical research. The National Council provided leadership in monitoring and promoting nurse and midwife involvement in research.[250] Nurses and midwives are involved in the management of these initiatives. Some of the new roles in the career pathway, including CNS/CMS and ANP/AMP, have built into their role description a requirement that they should lead in the development and application of clinical research in nursing and midwifery. In addition, the number of nurses who have pursued research leading to PhDs and doctoral and postdoctoral research in Ireland is increasing each year.

In 2006 the National Council published a report[251] that provides a picture of nursing and midwifery research activity in Ireland for the period 2002–2004. A number of proposed actions supported the recommendations of the *Research Strategy for Nursing and Midwifery in Ireland*.[252] Other recommendations were set out for building upon the baseline established by this project. A study to identify research priorities for nursing and midwifery in Ireland was carried out in 2005.[253] Key research topics included outcomes of care delivery, staffing issues, input into policy- and decision-making, and research-based practice. A second study, *Report on the Baseline Survey of Research Activity in Irish Nursing and Midwifery*,[254] was published by the National Council in 2006 and contained an overview of nursing and midwifery research carried out prior to the *Research Strategy*.[255] It therefore provided a baseline for future developments. In 2009, the Department of Health and Children published *Research Strategy for Nursing and Midwifery in Ireland 2003–2008: Review of Attainments*,[256] which provided a summary of the achievements in the area of research since the publication of the national strategy.

Joint Appointments

In 2005, the National Council published a report[257] on joint appointments that provided a framework for institutions and individuals involved in making joint appointments between services, voluntary organisations, educational institutions and/or other organisations. Joint appointments require careful planning and support mechanisms. The Commission on Nursing commissioned a special report on the use of joint appointments[258] and recommended that, in the transfer to a university/college-based degree programme, there should be a number of joint appointments between third-level institutes and health service providers. This report concluded that there appeared to be no single internationally recognised model for joint appointments. However, there were strong views in countries that had integrated pre-registration nursing education into the third-level sector that such appointments were essential to the success of the education programmes. These appointments involved a nurse combining an education role in a third-level institute with a clinical or research role within a health service provider.

Table 7 provides a general reference grid for current career pathways in nursing and midwifery, based on the recommendations contained in the *Report of the Commission on Nursing* and developments within the health services over the past fourteen years.

Table 7: Current Career Pathways in Nursing and Midwifery

Divisions of the Register	General nursing Midwifery Psychiatric nursing Intellectual disability nursing Children's nursing
Entry Qualification Required	Four-year honours degree
Role	Registered general nurse (RGN) Registered midwife (RM) Registered psychiatric nurse (RPN) Registered nurse intellectual disability (RNID) Registered children's nurse (RCN)
Role Progression (Clinical)	**Acute services:** Registered staff nurse/midwife Clinical nurse/midwife specialist (CNS/CMS) Advanced nurse/midwife practitioner (ANP/AMP) (Clinical nurse researcher)

(Continued)

Table 7: (*Continued*)

	Primary care: Registered nurse (general, psychiatric, intellectual disability, children's) Palliative nurse Registered midwife Public health nurse Practice nurse (Research)
Role Progression (Education)	**Third-level institutions:** College lecturer Statutory lecturer Senior lecturer Associate professor Professor (Research) **Centres for Nurse/Midwife Education (CNE/CME):** Clinical placement coordinator Practice development coordinator Tutor Director of CNE/CME (Research)
Role Progression (Management)	**Acute services:** Clinical nurse manager 1/clinical midwife manager 1 (CNM1/CMM1) Clinical nurse manager 2/clinical midwife manager 2 (CNM2/CMM2) Clinical nurse manager 3/clinical midwife manager 3 (CNM3/CMM3) Assistant director of nursing/midwifery or nurse/midwife manager Director of nursing/midwifery **Community-based services:** Assistant director of public health nursing Director of public health nursing
Joint Appointments	Clinical/academic joint appointments in nursing and midwifery

The changes introduced by the Commission on Nursing in relation to the clinical career pathway have led to a radical transformation of the professions. The first degree-qualified cohort of nurses/midwives emerged from the education system in 2006. There are now over 2,300 CNSs/CMSs and over 100 ANPs/AMPs in the health services.

Table 8: Clinical Specialists: Main Findings (Strong and Very Strong Evidence)

The clinical specialist's (CS) caseload involves working with the multidisciplinary team (MDT) to provide specialised assessment, planning, delivery and evaluation of care using protocol-driven guidelines. The CS role maximises the team impact on patient outcomes. Care delivery and caseload management is delivered in line with core concepts identified by the National Council (clinical focus, patient/client advocacy, education and training, audit and research, consultancy).

Clinical care is a significant part of the role of the CS in Ireland. This is contrary to international and, in particular, US profiles, where the literature shows CSs have limited patient/client contact. Overall, there was no additional cost for CS service (staff costs and activity levels for matched CS and non-CS services). CS services have decreased costs for colposcopy and managing challenging behaviour. CSs were working to expand and develop practice (many CSs were working towards an advanced practitioner (AP) role).

Box 1: Clinical Nurse Specialist, Main Findings (strong and very strong evidence)
Evidence demonstrated that CNSs:

- Reduced morbidity
- Decreased considerably service users' waiting times
- Provided earlier access to care (CNSs provided early access to first visits)
- Decreased readmission rates
- Increased evidence-based practice
- Increased use of clinical guidelines for MDT
- Increased continuity of care
- Increased patient/client satisfaction
- Increased communication with patients/clients and families
- Promoted patient/client self-management
- Had significant MDT support for the role
- Provided clinical leadership
- Conducted clinical audit (and 53% conducted research)

(Continued)

Table 8: (Continued)

Box 2: Clinical Midwife Specialist, Main Findings (strong and very strong evidence)
Evidence demonstrated that CMSs:

- Reduced morbidity
- Decreased waiting times
- Provided earlier access to care (CMSs provided earlier access to treatment)
- Decreased readmission rates
- Increased evidence-based practice
- Increased use of clinical guidelines for MDT
- Increased continuity of care (CMSs spent significant time with service users teaching, advising and explaining tests and results)
- Increased patient/client satisfaction (CMSs were noted by service users to make a difference to their care)
- Increased communication with patients/clients and families (CMSs spent significant time with service users discussing their problems)
- Promoted patient/client self-management
- Had significant MDT support for the role
- Provided clinical leadership
- Conducted clinical audit (and 53% conducted research)

The National Council published, in 2004, *An Evaluation of the Effectiveness of the Role of the Clinical Nurse/Midwife Specialist*,[259] which demonstrated that there was overwhelming support for the role of the CNS/CMS. In 2005 the National Council also published *A Preliminary Evaluation of the Role of the Advanced Nurse Practitioner*.[260] Although limited because of the size of the sample involved, this evaluation provided preliminary evidence that ANP roles enhanced patient/client care by providing a holistic service that improved their access to healthcare. The report also demonstrated that ANPs had been widely accepted by patients/clients, nurses, doctors and other members of the multidisciplinary team. There is an emerging body of evidence that underlines the positive impact of these changes. In 2010 the National Council published the results of a major two-year study,[261] *An Evaluation of the Role of the Clinical Nurse/Midwife Specialist and Advanced Nurse/Midwife Practitioner in Ireland*. The study concluded that the research has demonstrated conclusively that care provided by CNSs/CMSs and ANPs/AMPs improved patient/client outcomes, was safe, acceptable and cost neutral.[262] The main findings are summarised in the Tables 8 and 9, which include extracts from the final report.[263] The study also suggests that ANPs/AMPs do give a higher level of care, particularly at a strategic level. It concludes that existing CNSs/CMSs should be encouraged to develop their skills and education to achieve advanced practice level and that more specialist and advanced practice posts should be created.[264]

**Table 9: Advanced Practitioners (AP):
Main Findings (Strong and Very Strong Evidence)**

The AP caseload involves holistic assessment, diagnosis, autonomous decision-making regarding treatment, provision of interventions and discharge from a full episode of care. Care delivery and caseload management is provided by APs in line with core concepts identified by the National Council (autonomy in clinical practice, expert practice, professional and clinical leadership, research).

The education level of APs in Ireland is in line with international standards. Overall, there was no additional costs for AP services (staff costs and activity levels for matched AP and non-AP services). AP services had decreased costs for emergency department minor injuries and sexual health.

(Continued)

Table 9: (*Continued*)

Box 3: Clinical Nurse Specialist, Main Findings (strong and very strong evidence)

Evidence demonstrated that CNSs:

- Reduced morbidity
- Decreased waiting times
- Provided earlier access to care
- Decreased readmission rates
- Increased patient/client throughput
- Increased evidence-based practice
- Increased use of clinical guidelines for MDT
- Developed guidelines for local, regional and national distribution
- Increased continuity of care
- Increased patient/client satisfaction
- Increased communication with patients/clients and families
- Promoted patient/client self-management
- Worked to expand and develop scope of practice to include more complex care provision
- Demonstrated high job satisfaction
- Had significant MDT support for the role
- Provided clinical and professional leadership
- Conducted audits and research

Strategic Framework for Role Expansion of Nurses and Midwives

Nurses and midwives have in recent times been required to extend and expand their practice in order to respond to the needs of the services and of the patients/clients they serve. Examples of this include implementing the clinical career pathway and introducing specialisation at the level of CNS/CMS and ANP/AMP, expanding scope of practice through nurse- and midwife-led services, the introduction of prescribing of medication and ionising radiation for nurses and midwives, and expanded clinical decision-making in both acute and community settings. As the health services develop in Ireland in line with developing Government policy and the requirements of the services, nurses and midwives will continue to provide high-quality, responsive care with enhanced roles reflecting their education, CPD and expertise into the future. This care will be provided in acute and community settings and in roles that span the boundaries of both. The roles will develop for acute and chronic illnesses, palliative care and across the lifespan of the patients and clients of the services.

This requirement poses a challenge to individual nurses and midwives and to those responsible for ensuring that services are delivered in a manner that is safe and protects the public. The first reference point that nurses and midwives turn to for guidance in responding to the demands for extension and expansion of practice is that provided by An Bord Altranais. This is contained in the guidance provided by An Bord Altranais on practice and on competencies required to practice and is further made explicit in the Scope of Practice Framework[265] and the Code of Professional Conduct.[266] Further guidance is provided by the criteria for specialist and advanced practice that were produced by the National Council. The scope of nursing and midwifery practice in Ireland is defined by An Bord Altranais as the range of roles, functions, responsibilities and activities that a registered nurse or midwife is educated, competent and has authority to perform.[267]

The publication by the Department of Health of the *Strategic Framework for Role Expansion of Nurses and Midwives: Promoting Quality Patient Care*[268] has provided policy direction outlining the process for successful consideration of expansion of nursing and midwifery practice. This framework describes a six-step process that should be followed in determining whether an expansion of role and practice should be considered and, if so, what considerations should be taken into account in proceeding with the expansion.

The framework states that the decision on whether to expand nurses' or midwives' roles should be based on a service needs analysis and an assessment of the skill mix that is available. The National Council's *Service Needs Analysis: Informing Business and Service Plans*[269] outlined a service needs analysis process which gives consideration to population health, epidemiology, workforce planning, HSE requirements, new ways of working and developing a business case. Additionally, *Improving the Patient Journey: Understanding Integrated Care Pathways*[270] provides guidance in relation to patient process mapping, which can assist in identifying gaps in patient service delivery.

Once the decision has been taken, the framework states that an examination of the impact on service delivery should be carried out. This is based on the principle that the decision to expand practice should be based on improving the patient journey through the service. Analysis of the impact on service delivery therefore should consider issues such as the impact on skill mix, the patient journey, anticipated patient outcomes and available resources.

The considerations that should be taken into account in deciding to expand the roles include a review of the *Scope of Nursing and Midwifery Practice Framework;*[271] determining the responsibilities associated with the expanded role; assessing the required level of expertise and clinical decision-making that is required in the expanded role (i.e. is the role appropriate for a staff nurse/midwife, CNS/CMS or ANP/AMP?);[272] determining the competencies that are required for the role; identifying the relevant guidelines, policies and protocols that must be taken into account;[273] and, finally, sourcing the required clinical and professional leadership.

The final step in the framework is the evaluation of the clinical outcomes[274] that the expanded roles set out to achieve in order to assess the impact of the expansion of the roles of nurses and midwives.

Enhanced nursing and midwifery roles are of critical importance in supporting the implementation of the national clinical programmes and the cancer control programme referred to in Chapter 2 of this book. Development and expansion of nursing and midwifery practice increasingly takes place in the context of multidisciplinary, multi-skilled teams. National, regional and local guidelines, protocols and frameworks provide the standards required for best practice by all members of the multidisciplinary team.

The extent of expanded and enhanced care provision being provided by general nurses is illustrated in the case studies provided in the *Strategic Framework for Role Expansion of Nurses and Midwives: Promoting Quality Patient Care.*[275] The examples include the roles that ANPs are developing within the services (e.g. ANP-led services in emergency departments, diabetes and cardiology); the application and care of continuous positive airway pressure (CPAP), bilevel positive airway pressure (BiPAP) and non-invasive ventilation (NIV); the roles that CNSs are developing within the services (e.g. diabetes, COPD, heart failure); electrocardiogram analysis; follow-up clinics for older person services (e.g. dementia, Parkinson's disease); ionising radiation prescribing; intravenous cannulation and venepuncture; male catheterisation; medication prescribing; nurse-led clinics (e.g. leg ulcer clinics); nurse-led discharge utilising agreed protocols; and pre-operative assessment.

Midwifery-led care has long been an aspiration of midwives and women in Ireland.[276] The *Report of the Maternity Review Group* in the former North Eastern Health Board (NEHB) proposed the setting up of two midwife-led units attached to conventional maternity units in the NEHB.[277] Many midwives have stated that they are now actively seeking opportunities to practise midwifery within settings that provide midwives with autonomy and pregnant women with alternative choices in childbirth.[278] There are examples of innovative community practice taking place at present, such as the service provided by the Southern Health Area (SHA), which employs independent midwives to provide domiciliary maternity services. The evaluation of the pilot scheme DOMINO (domiciliary care in and out of hospital) in the National Maternity Hospital showed that it was extremely successful and viable and, given sufficient funding, was sustainable in the long term.[279] The evaluation made a strong case for the development of similar schemes in other Dublin maternity hospitals and in maternity units around the country.

Examples of expanded roles for midwives include midwife-led discharges; midwife-led pre-booking clinic at twelve weeks gestation; midwives' clinics for low-risk women throughout pregnancy; midwife-led diabetic clinics; bereavement and miscarriage clinics; roles being developed by CMSs (e.g. diabetes, drugs liaison, bereavement and loss); counselling and psychological care; domestic abuse screening; drop-in clinics; examination of the newborn; helpline service for mothers and professionals; increased community services and outreach clinics; ultrasonography services (e.g. foetal assessment, antenatal diagnosis, foetal therapy and associated counselling and management); roles being developed by AMPs (e.g. diabetes: continuity of care for women with Type 1, Type 2 and gestational diabetes; AMP neonatal: admissions, newborn assessment, ordering investigations, interpretation of results, central catheter placement, IV cannulation, referrals, prescribing, resuscitation, intubation and transport; AMP urodynamics: comprehensive health assessment, plans and initiating care and treatment modalities to achieve patient-centred outcomes and evaluate their effectiveness, initiating and terminating a care episode within the agreed scope of AMP practice guidelines; AMP caseload management: provision of clinical supervision, leadership).

The Strategic Framework[280] also contains case studies of expansion of practice within the disciplines of intellectual disability nursing, psychiatric nursing and children's nursing.

CHAPTER 6

Nursing and Midwifery in the Irish Health Services

The Nursing and Midwifery Resource

In order to appreciate the scale of the nursing and midwifery contribution to the Irish health services, it is important to consider the latest information on the overall composition of the workforce in healthcare in Ireland. Table 10 provides an overview for the years 2002, 2010 and 2011.[281]

Table 10: Employment in the Public Health Services by Category, 2002, 2010, 2011

Grade Category	2002	2010	2011*	% Change	
				2002–2011	2010–2011
Medical/dental	6,775	8,096	8,142	20.2%	0.6%
General support staff	13,729	11,421	10,652	−22.4%	−6.7%
Health and social care professionals	12,577	16,355	16,165	28.5%	−1.2%
Management/ administration	15,690	17,301	16,058	2.3%	−7.2%
Other patient and client care	13,513	18,295	17,276	27.8%	−5.6%
Nursing	33,395	36,503	35,993	7.8%	−1.4%
Total	95,679	107,971	104,286	9.0%	−3.4%

As can be seen, the largest group by far in the table is nursing.[282] Most of the groups have experienced increases in their numbers for the period 2002–2011, with the exception of general support staff, which recorded a decrease of 22.4 per cent over the ten-year period. When one looks at the data for the period 2010–2011 (covering the period of the bailout and the austerity measures in public expenditure), all the groups, with the exception of medical/dental, experienced reductions.

Table 11 looks at the percentage breakdown by category for the year 2011. Nursing and midwifery make up just over one-third of the healthcare workforce.

Table 11: Employment in the Public Health Services by Category, 2011

Grade Category	2011	Percentage
Medical/dental	8,142	7.8%
General support staff	10,652	10.2%
Health and social care professionals	16,165	15.5%
Management/administration	16,058	15.4%
Other patient and client care	17,276	16.6%
Nursing	35,993	34.5%
Total	**104,286**	**100.0%**

If one excludes general support staff, management and administration and considers only those who are directly involved in the provision of care to patients and clients, nurses and midwives make up over 46 per cent of the workforce (see Table 12). However, when one considers the role of nursing and midwifery as being a coordinator of care and having responsibility for the inputs of those referred to as 'other patient and client care' personnel (including healthcare assistants, porters and emergency medical technicians), the professions are responsible for over two-thirds (68.7 per cent) of the care providers within the health services. In addition, the involvement of nurses and midwives in care delivery requires them to be in direct contact with patients and clients 24 hours a day, seven days a week. This marks them out from all other professionals in terms of their impact on service delivery. They are also frequently directly responsible for the coordination and management of the inputs of the health and social care professionals in both acute and primary care settings.

Table 12: Employment in the Public Health Services by Category, 2011 (Excluding Management and Administrative and General Support Staff)

Grade Category	2011	Percentage
Medical/dental	8,142	10.5%
Health and social care professionals	16,165	20.8%
Other patient and client care	17,276	22.3%
Nursing	35,993	46.4%
Total	77,576	100.0%

Nursing and midwifery are the lynchpins in the delivery of health services in Ireland because of the pervasive nature of their role, the scale of their presence and the central position they occupy on behalf of the patient or client. The scale of the nursing and midwifery presence within the health services carries with it a heavy duty of responsibility to fulfil that professional role at all times in the best interests of the patients and clients of the service. Nurses and midwives are not just another group of employees among the more than 104,000 employees of the health services. They are the bulwark, the platform and the principal conduit through which care is provided to vulnerable and dependent patients and clients.

Health Service Challenges for Nursing and Midwifery

The professions face many new and complex challenges within the health services in the context of the reform programmes and policy priorities contained in the Programme for Government and the challenges contained in a wide range of other key healthcare strategy and policy documents.

Chronic Diseases

In line with international trends in developed countries, the demographic and epidemiological profile of the Irish population is changing. Ireland ranks among the high-income developed countries of Europe and, in common with others, Irish people are living longer. Chronic diseases, including cancers, according to a 2010 WHO study,[283] account for the majority of deaths and diseases in Europe. The study estimated that in 2005 chronic or non-communicable conditions accounted for 86 per cent of deaths in the

European region and that 72 per cent of all deaths before the age of 60 years were due to chronic or non-communicable diseases in high-income countries. This would suggest that chronic disease can no longer be considered just a problem of the elderly.

In addition to looking at the causes of deaths, the WHO study also looked at the burden of disease. This is usually expressed in terms of a disability-adjusted life year (DALY), which is designed to quantify the impact on a population of premature death and disability by combining them into one single measure. The DALY is based on the assumption that the most appropriate measure of the effects of chronic illness is time spent either disabled by the disease or lost due to premature death. With this measure, one DALY equals one year of healthy life lost.[284] Using this measure, chronic or non-communicable diseases are estimated to account for 77 per cent of the total burden of disease in the European region in 2005.

Chronic diseases include cardiovascular disease, diabetes, and asthma/COPD. More recently, as survival rates and treatments have improved, they also include many varieties of cancer, HIV/AIDS, mental disorders (such as depression, schizophrenia and dementia) and disabilities such as sight impairment and arthroses. Many chronic diseases and conditions are linked to an ageing society, but also to lifestyle choices such as smoking, sexual behaviour, diet and exercise, as well as to genetic predispositions.[285]

All of these diseases require long-term and complex responses involving different healthcare professionals with access to the necessary drugs and equipment. The responses extend beyond healthcare into wider social care interventions, crossing over a range of disciplines. In order to provide this kind of care, it is necessary to move beyond the traditional structures of healthcare provision that have been dominated by 'acute' interventions in hospitals. It is also necessary to move beyond the traditional demarcation lines between the professions towards a more integrated approach involving the emergence of new providers, new care settings and, as a consequence, new qualifications in those providing the care.

Many countries throughout Europe, including Ireland, have developed chronic disease management programmes that aim to improve chronic care, contain costs, improve coordination, focusing on the whole care process, and build on scientific evidence and patient involvement. The roles of the general nurse, the CNS and the ANP are critical for the success of these programmes. For the programmes to be successful, they require the building of collaborative models, including the provision of nurse-led clinics that span acute hospital and community care settings. The WHO study[286] noted that evidence from pilot studies suggested that primary care nurses with more qualifications and responsibilities provided better care.

In Ireland, the Irish Hospice Foundation and the HSE conducted a joint study in 2007/2008 on extending access to palliative care for people with chronic diseases other than cancer and other life-threatening diseases.[287] The terms of reference of the study were to examine the palliative care needs of people with life-limiting diseases other than cancer, with an initial emphasis on dementia, COPD and heart failure, and to identify how the palliative model of care could be applied to these patient groups within the Irish healthcare context. The report on the study – *Palliative Care for All: Integrating Palliative Care into Disease Management Frameworks* – was published in December 2008. The report made overarching recommendations in relation to the development of policy, education, service models and research, as well as specific recommendations in relation to palliative care and dementia, palliative care and COPD, and palliative care and heart failure.

The National Clinical Programmes

In Ireland, the national clinical programmes,[288] which are an important part of the Government's health strategy as outlined in the Programme for Government,[289] were originally set up by the HSE's quality and clinical care directorate (QCCD). In December 2011, the directorate moved into the Department of Health as part of the reforms provided for in the Programme for Government. The national clinical programmes were established to improve and standardise patient care by bringing together clinical disciplines and enabling them to share innovative solutions to deliver greater benefits to every user of the health services. The objectives of the programmes are to improve the quality of care delivered to all users of healthcare services, to improve access to all services and to improve cost-effectiveness.

Table 13 lists the current national clinical programmes. These programmes define the clinical environment within which nurses and midwives will be working in Ireland for the foreseeable future and include many of the key chronic diseases referred to earlier.

Table 13: National Clinical Programmes

National Clinical Programmes (HSE 2012)[290]	
Acute Coronary Syndrome	Heart Failure
Acute Medicine	Medicines Management and Pharmacotherapeutic Interventions
Asthma	Obstetrics and Gynaecology
Audiology	Orthopaedics
Blood Transfusion	Outpatient Parenteral Antimicrobial Therapy (OPAT)
Care of the Elderly	Palliative Care
Chronic Obstructive Pulmonary Disease (COPD)	Prevention of Healthcare-Associated Infection (HCAI) and Antimicrobial Resistance (AMR)
Critical Care	Primary Care
Dermatology	Radiology
Diabetes	Rehabilitation Medicine
Elective Surgery (ESP)	Renal
Emergency Medicine (EMP)	Rheumatology
Epilepsy	Stroke

One of the first national clinical programmes to be developed was the national acute medicine programme. It is a good example of the way in which these programmes work and the key role that nursing is expected to play in achieving their objectives.

The Programme for Government 2011 commits to reforming the model of delivering healthcare, so that more care is delivered in the community. The aim of primary and community care services is to support and promote the health and well-being of the population by making people's first point of contact with the health services easily accessible, integrated and locally based. As services move to community settings, acute inpatient care has intensified, with shorter hospital stays, increased use of technology and non-invasive treatments creating a higher mix of patient acuity. This has been evidenced by the usage statistics published in *Health in Ireland: Key Trends 2011*, summarised in Chapter 2 of this book.

The national acute medicine programme is a clinician-led initiative between the Royal College of Physicians of Ireland, the

Irish Association of Directors of Nursing and Midwifery, the Therapy Professions Committee, the Irish College of General Practitioners and the QCCD. The programme recognises the essential role of large and small hospitals, GPs and community services. It provides a framework for the delivery of acute medical services which seeks to substantially improve patient care.

The *Report of the National Acute Medicine Programme*[291] provides a framework for acute medical care. The aim of the programme is the standardisation of access to and delivery of high-quality, safe acute medicine services nationally. The programme proposes that there should be four levels of acute hospitals for acute medicine patients:

- Model 4: tertiary hospitals are usually major hospitals with a full complement of services including paediatrics, obstetrics, general medicine, gynaecology, various branches of surgery and psychiatry or a speciality hospital dedicated to specific sub-speciality care (paediatric centres, oncology centres, psychiatric hospitals). Patients will often be referred from smaller hospitals to a tertiary hospital for major operations, consultations with sub-specialists and when sophisticated intensive care facilities are required.
- Model 3: general hospitals are usually large hospitals set up to deal with many kinds of disease and injury, and normally have an emergency department to deal with immediate and urgent threats to health.
- Model 2: local hospitals, with selected (GP-referred) medical patients
- Model 1: community/district hospitals

The report indicates that the future growth in healthcare will be in ambulatory care provided across the acute–primary care–community interface. This will include chronic disease management, day surgery, diagnostics and rehabilitation. Much of this will be based in local (Model 2) hospitals. The programme aims to establish navigation hubs incorporating bed managers and case managers. These hubs will be developed in the context of an integrated service area (ISA) and will support the streaming of patients referred by GPs to the most appropriate available care setting. This will help enhance communication between primary care, community services and hospital-based services. The programme also proposes that acute medical patients should be managed in dedicated acute medical units (AMUs) (located in Model 4 tertiary hospitals), acute medical assessment units (AMAUs) (located in Model 3 general hospitals) and medical assessment units (MAUs) (located in Model 2 local hospitals) and that timely care from a senior medical doctor will be provided when needed.

The report states that the director of nursing, assistant director of nursing, divisional nurse managers, CNMs and nursing staff should have a role in the strategic development of these units. CNMs in particular have a crucial role in ensuring the success of the AMU/AMAU/MAU. The CNMs and nursing staff are responsible for the day-to-day management and will also support the strategic development of the unit, implement policies and ensure robust systems are in place for the admission, handover and discharge of patients, ensuring that there are effective links with GPs, carers and other relevant community services. They are also expected to provide leadership and ensure efficient and effective communication with patients and relatives, other health-care providers and multidisciplinary team members. The CNM is expected to place particular emphasis on ensuring the timely initiation of patient assessment, instigation of safe care and completion of unit care – whether by handover to another hospital unit/service or GP/community service. CNMs in relevant chronic disease fields will make an important contribution to patient care in the AMU/AMAU/MAU. In addition to core AMU/AMAU/MAU nursing staff, the development of CNS and ANP posts specialising in acute medicine is recommended incorporating skill sets and competency development. Particular emphasis on independent assessment and development of initial treatment plans by specialist and advanced practice nurses is recommended.

An important complement to the national acute medicine programme is the emergency medicine programme. The *National Emergency Medicine Programme*[292] (EMP) was published in June 2012, after extensive consultation with patients and front-line staff across the health services. The programme, which has been developed by doctors, nurses, therapists and other clinicians working in emergency departments and in pre-hospital care, sets out an ambitious programme of reform for how emergency services are delivered in Ireland. The aim of the emergency medicine programme is to improve the safety and quality of care and to reduce waiting times for patients in emergency departments. The EMP is a blueprint for the future development of emergency care in Ireland. It sets out an unprecedented, ambitious programme of work that includes the development of new models of care for the treatment of patients, expanding the roles of nurses and increasing the level of consultant-provided care. The programme also sets out to improve ED efficiency and to implement new clinical guidelines in emergency care.

Cancer Care

The *Strategy for Cancer Control in Ireland*[293] provides the policy direction for the treatment and control of cancer in Ireland. The strategy was published in 2006 and was the second national cancer strategy. It focused substantially on reform and reorganisation of the way cancer services were delivered in order to ensure that future services would be consistent and associated with a high-quality experience for patients and their carers. The strategy advocates a comprehensive cancer control policy programme, which it defines as a whole-population, integrated and cohesive approach to cancer that involves prevention, screening, diagnosis, treatment, and supportive and palliative care. It places a major emphasis on measurement of need and on addressing inequalities and implies the need to focus on ensuring that all elements of cancer policy and service are delivered to the maximum possible extent.

The HSE's national cancer control programme (HSE-NCCP) was established in 2007 to reorganise cancer services to achieve better outcomes for patients. Under the programme, there are four designated cancer control networks and eight cancer centres nationally.[294] The four networks are HSE Dublin – North East; HSE Dublin – Mid Leinster; HSE South; and HSE West. The eight cancer centres are Beaumont Hospital, Mater Misericordiae University Hospital, St James's Hospital, St Vincent's University Hospital, Cork University Hospital, Waterford Regional Hospital, University College Hospital Galway (with a satellite in Letterkenny) and Limerick Regional Hospital. The programme is working to ensure that designated cancer centres for individual tumour types have adequate case volumes, expertise and concentration of multidisciplinary specialist skills.

The most recent *National Cancer Control Programme Fact Sheet*[295] reports that 24,800 new cases of invasive cancers are diagnosed each year in Ireland. The number of new cases being diagnosed each year is rising by over 6 per cent per annum and is projected to reach

55,000 by the year 2030. There have been dramatic rises in the survival rates for cancers. Five-year survival rates improved from 40 per cent in 1994 to 55 per cent for the period 2004 to 2007. The fact sheet states that 30 per cent of cancer cases could be prevented, mainly by not smoking and introducing changes in lifestyle.

To date, the programme has reorganised all breast cancer diagnostic and surgical services into the eight cancer centres only (plus an outreach service in Letterkenny General Hospital); established rapid access diagnostic clinics for prostate cancer and lung cancer in all eight cancer centres; established a national centre for pancreatic cancer surgery; centralised all lung surgery into four cancer centres; developed a national service for ocular cancer; developed a single national programme (operating on two sites) for the management of brain tumours and other central nervous system tumours; developed national GP referral guidelines and standard referral forms for breast, lung and prostate cancers, making the referral process more seamless, safer and more efficient; and developed electronic cancer referral for breast, prostate and lung cancer in collaboration with a broad range of stakeholders, which ensures rapid referral of patients with suspected cancer in a secure manner.

The programme has developed a community oncology nurse programme, an initiative aimed at integrating medical oncology care between the acute hospital and community settings. It has also developed and implemented a training programme for nurses who work in primary care, with a particular focus on practice nurses. This course covers cancer prevention, referral and patient assessment, treatment and post-acute care.

New radiation oncology facilities at St James's Hospital and Beaumont Hospital were completed and opened under Phase 1 of the national plan for radiation oncology in 2011. The new centres reflect the latest advances, equipment and expertise available internationally and deliver an increase of 50 per cent in the number of linear accelerators in the eastern region (from eight to twelve). For patients, this means improved access, the most advanced technology, increased professional staffing levels and a revised pathway, so that they will now start treatment significantly quicker than before, and in line with the best international standards. The Irish Government has committed to making a significant capital contribution to the provision of a satellite centre for radiation oncology in Altnagelvin Hospital, linked to Belfast City Hospital. This contribution recognises the fact that approximately one-third of the patients who will attend the proposed Altnagelvin Centre will be from Donegal and surrounding areas.

CervicalCheck provides free smear tests to women aged 25 to 60. In 2010, over 329,000 women were screened. BreastCheck provides free mammograms to all women aged 50–64 and is now available nationwide. In 2010, over 118,800 women were screened. A colorectal screening programme, set to start on a national basis in late 2012, will initially target people aged between 60 and 69. Free screening will be offered to 400,000 people in this age group. The programme will be extended to all those aged 55 to 74 years of age as resources allow. The national human papillomavirus (HPV) vaccination programme commenced in 2010. The vaccine is now offered to all girls in first year in secondary school (aged about 13) each year. A catch-up programme for girls in sixth year of secondary school (aged about 18) commenced in September 2011 and will continue for sixth-year girls in 2012 and 2013.

Maternity

As noted in Chapter 2 of this book, the number of births in 2010 – at 73,724 – is about 15,000 more births annually than a decade ago.[296] This increased birth rate has led to an increase in demand for maternity services. Pregnant women want a wide range of choices when it comes to models of maternity care. A recent survey[297] indicated that 46 per cent would prefer to have their baby delivered in a doctor-led unit and 43 per cent in a midwifery-led unit, with choice strongly influenced by safety considerations. A number of important reports, strategies and policy documents have been produced in recent years that are shaping the way in which maternity and gynaecological services will be delivered in Ireland.

A detailed review of all maternity services in the greater Dublin area was commissioned in 2007 by the HSE. The contract to conduct the review was awarded to KPMG, who published their report in 2008 entitled *Independent Review of Maternity and Gynaecology Services in the Greater Dublin Area*.[298] The purposes of the review were to build on the strengths of the current service configuration and model of care; to define the optimal configuration of maternity, gynaecology and neonatology services for the greater Dublin area; to identify the optimal location of services; and to provide a roadmap for the future, outlining the steps required to get from where the service was then to a vision for the future.

According to the review, by international standards the current maternity service model in Ireland was relatively hospital-focused, with a strong emphasis on medically led services, and this model had been largely defined by the provisions of the Mother and Infant Scheme,[299] which provides for free medical care for expectant mothers and their newly born babies as provided by their family GP and a hospital-based obstetrician. There did not exist at the time within the model of service delivery an option for midwifery-led care. As a result, midwifery-led or midwifery-delivered services were relatively underdeveloped. The review also said that the structure of private medical insurance also played a key role in maintaining doctor-led services.

Despite the fact that the current model of care favours GP involvement over that of midwives, primary-care-based services are underdeveloped to deliver it. Primary care in Ireland as a whole is underdeveloped and this is evident in a lack of community maternity and gynaecology services. Services that are available tend to be outreach services from the hospital rather than provided by primary, community and continuing care (PCCC). The dominance of a medically led, hospital-centred model of care provides effective services for women with non-routine clinical conditions. However, approximately 60 per cent of women experience a normal pregnancy and birth. It does therefore limit the choice for women whose routine clinical needs could be provided for in a wider range of settings.[300]

The review contained a number of long-term recommendations in relation to the development of suitable medical infrastructure. In the short term, however, prior to any investment, the review recommended a number of measures that would serve to significantly enhance the quality of existing services. These measures included[301] addressing the performance improvement opportunities around metrics like 'did not attend' rates, average length of stay, bed/theatre capacity management, caesarean section rates, day-case rates for gynaecology, workforce numbers, etc; developing an education and training programme for midwives and GPs around the various alternatives to giving birth in hospital, supported by a public PR campaign and debate around the fact that these represent safe alternatives to hospital birth; developing multidisciplinary teams for socially excluded women for antenatal care and follow-up; and developing an education and training programme for GPs aimed at ensuring that women are referred from primary into secondary gynaecological care using integrated pathways.

The review saw a need for structures that would facilitate the enhancement of team-working and allow for the seamless coordinated movement of women and/or their babies, regardless of the level of care required. The review emphasised the need to strengthen community care and recommended that the current DOMINO scheme, where a women receives antenatal care delivered by community-based midwives close to the woman's home, should be extended to cover 20 per cent of women; it also recommended the strengthening of outreach and early transfer home schemes, which should be significantly expanded to provide antenatal care in the community for all women who are assessed as low risk. The review also proposed that all women should have access to efficient and effective community-based, midwife-provided postnatal care.

In 2005, the HSE produced a strategy for the maternity services in the eastern region entitled *Maternity Services in the Eastern Region: A Strategy for the Future, 2005–2011*.[302] The strategy stated that there is a need for services to be provided through a range of service initiatives and a variety of models of care, in order to enhance the quality of care and provide women with choice. Key recommendations within the report included an interdisciplinary team approach to the maternity services across all levels of care; continued development of community-based maternity services for women with low-risk pregnancies; services to continue to be responsive to the needs of vulnerable and disadvantaged women; and the development and implementation of models of care within and between primary and secondary care to increase choice and continuity of care for women.

Recent Irish research provides evidence that midwifery-led care is as safe as consultant-led care. The report of the MidU Study (Midwifery-Led Unit Study),[303] carried out between 2004 and 2007, was a pragmatic two-group randomised controlled trial comparing midwifery-led care provided for low-risk women in an integrated midwifery-led unit (MLU) using evidence-based policies and procedural guidelines, with consultant-led care, in the HSE north-eastern region. The results have shown that midwifery-led care, as practised in this study, is as safe as consultant-led care, results in less intervention, is viewed by women with greater satisfaction in some aspects of care and is more cost-effective.[304] These results compare favourably to international research on midwife-led care,[305] which also presents evidence supporting the policy of offering low-risk women a choice of birth setting.

The Institute of Obstetricians and Gynaecologists, in its report *The Future of Maternity and Gynaecology Services in Ireland 2006–2016*,[306] addresses the need for the integration of primary and secondary care within the maternity services. It recognises the crucial role that midwives play in pregnancy and particularly in relation to 'normal' pregnancies and supports the expansion of the DOMINO service nationally and the development of new career paths for midwifery, including further development of CMSs and AMPs.

The *Strategic Framework for Role Expansion of Nurses and Midwives*,[307] discussed in Chapter 5, refers to a number of expanded and enhanced roles for midwives. In addition to care of low-risk women, midwives are managing the wider complex health needs of women and babies.

The report of *The Lourdes Hospital Inquiry*[308] made a number of recommendations that have implications for midwifery care. It found that support systems must be in place to conduct regular and obligatory audits and that there must be mandatory CPD and skills assessment at all levels of healthcare. Staff also need to attend regular programmes aimed at updating skills and competencies (this is now mandatory following the enactment of the Nurses and Midwives Act 2011, which provides for mandatory maintenance of professional competence by all nurses and midwives) and should be able to recognise that procedures change in accordance with evidence-based research.

The national clinical programme for obstetrics and gynaecology[309] has as its stated aim the improvement of choice in women's healthcare. In order to do this, it aims to increase the number of patients attending for antenatal care in early pregnancy from 55 per cent of total births in 2007 to 70 per cent in 2012. It aims to improve choice by developing and delivering new models of maternity care.

It is important to acknowledge the significant developments that have taken place in midwifery care in Ireland. Recent developments and new models of care have resulted in the provision of greater choice for women. These include the DOMINO schemes, examination of the newborn, increased community services and midwifery-led units. The policy direction for maternity care is developing in a way that will enhance the role of the midwife, the CMS and AMP within the health service so that it promotes a holistic support approach to the provision of care, adequately supported when required by appropriate medical interventions. This is the environment in which the midwife of the future will be working in Ireland.

Mental Health

There are many challenges facing nurses who are involved in the provision of mental health services in Ireland today. Mental health policy will be a key driver in determining the environment for psychiatric nursing practice. A significant volume of care will be delivered in community settings and many of the traditional mental health institutions have either already closed or will close in the near future. Psychiatric nurse graduates will be practising in line with these trends in mental healthcare delivery.

The Programme for Government 2011[310] contains commitments to a comprehensive range of mental health services as part of the standard insurance package offered under the UHI scheme that the Government proposes to introduce. The Programme endorses the content and aims of the key policy document *A Vision for Change* and is committed to the development of community mental health teams and services, as outlined in *A Vision for Change*, in order to ensure early access to more appropriate services for adults and children and improved integration with primary care services. The Government also stated that it intended to review the Mental Health Act 2001[311] in consultation with service users, carers and other stakeholders and informed by human rights standards. A Mental Capacity Bill that is in line with the UN Convention on the Rights of Persons with Disabilities[312] would also be introduced.

In 2012 the Minister for Disability, Equality, Mental Health and Older People published the *Interim Report of the Steering Group on the Review of the Mental Health Act 2001*[313] in part fulfilment of the commitment contained in the Programme for Government. The steering group recommended that a rights-based approach to mental health law should be adopted. It reported that, during the consultation process, strong views were expressed that there should be a move away from the paternalistic approach of the 2001 Act. The interim report stated that each person should have the right to determine and participate as much as they possibly could in their own care and treatment and the imminent publication of the Assisted Decision-Making (Capacity) Bill 2012[314] would be important progress in this regard. The interim report also emphasised the need for revised mental health legislation to support the objectives of *A Vision for Change*, especially in relation to the promotion of community-based mental health services. The interim report also made recommendations aimed at improving procedures regarding the detention of individuals and the necessary safeguards needed to ensure that they received the maximum appropriate protection. It also recommended that provisions relating to children should be included in a standalone part of the Act and that children should be given a greater say in their care and treatment. The Minister, in welcoming the report, indicated her intention to put in place an expert group to carry out the second and substantive phase of the review. She indicated that this group would begin its work during the second half of 2012 and would conclude its deliberations in early 2013.[315]

Much progress has already been made in mental health services since the publication of the first major strategy, *Planning for the Future*,[316] in 1984, which recommended a radical change in the way in which mental health services were delivered and a shift towards community-based care.

In 2006 *A Vision for Change: Report of the Expert Group on Mental Health Policy*[317] recommended additional fundamental changes in the way services were delivered and in the development of the infrastructure that would be required to support these changes. The report recommended that there should be greater involvement of service users and their carers and this should be a feature of every aspect of service development and delivery; mental health promotion should be available for all age groups, to enhance protective factors and decrease risk factors for developing mental health problems; well-trained, fully staffed, community-based, multidisciplinary community mental health teams (CMHTs) should be put in place for all mental health services. These teams should provide mental health services across an individual's lifespan. In order to be able to provide an effective community-based service, CMHTs should offer multidisciplinary home-based and assertive outreach care, and a comprehensive range of medical, psychological and social therapies relevant to the needs of service users and their families.

The report[318] also recommended that a recovery orientation should inform every aspect of service delivery and service users should be partners in their own care. Care plans should reflect the service user's particular needs, goals and potential and should address community factors that may impede or support recovery.

Links between specialist mental health services, primary care services and voluntary groups that are supportive of mental health should be enhanced and formalised. Services should be evaluated with meaningful performance indicators annually to assess the added value the service is contributing to the mental health of the local catchment area population.

The report recommended that all mental hospitals be closed and the resources released should be reinvested in the mental health service. Mental health information systems should be developed locally and should provide the national minimum mental health data set to a central mental health information system. Broadly based mental health service research should be undertaken and funded. Planning and funding of education and training for mental health professionals should be centralised in the new structures to be established by the HSE. A multi-professional manpower plan should be put in place, linked to projected service plans. This plan should look at the skill mix of teams and the way staff are deployed between teams and geographically, taking into account the service models recommended in the report. This plan should be prepared by the national mental health service directorate, working closely with the HSE, the Department of Health and Children and service providers.

In 2012 the Office of the Nursing and Midwifery Services Director of the HSE published *A Vision for Psychiatric/Mental Health Nursing: A Shared Journey for Mental Health Care in Ireland*[319] as a direct response to the *Vision for Change*[320] report. The report is the first formal strategy for psychiatric/mental health nursing in Ireland. It aims to provide guidance for nurses on the implementation of the recovery approach advocated by *A Vision for Change* and identifying what is required in order to ensure that this is embedded in clinical practice for the benefit of service users.

The HSE's QCCD appointed a national clinical programme director for mental health in 2010 with the stated aim of introducing evidence-based and standardised clinical pathways for specific mental health issues. Multidisciplinary working groups have been established to design the care pathway with service users. Initial priority programme design has commenced in the early identification of psychosis, self-harm and suicide, eating disorders, physical health needs of people with enduring mental illness, delirium and recovery.[321]

The Mental Health Commission was established in 2002 to promote, encourage and foster the establishment and maintenance of high standards and good practice in the delivery of mental health services. The annual reports of the inspector of mental health services are important indicators of the quality of the mental health services and provide recommendations for service development. The Mental Health Commission's *Annual Report for 2011* was published in April 2012 and included the report of the inspector of mental health services.[322] The report contains information on the continued winding-down of the old mental hospitals, the active involvement of service users in their care and treatment plans and the decrease in 2010 and again in 2011 in the number of child admissions to adult units. The report states that additional child and adolescent beds have been provided in Cork, Dublin and Galway. These beds, together with the Commission's Code of Practice on the Admission of Children under the Mental Health Act, 2001, which prohibits the admission of young people under eighteen years to adult units from 1 December 2011 (except in very exceptional circumstances), will greatly reduce and ultimately eliminate the inappropriate admission of children and young people to adult services.

In launching the report, the Minister for Health reiterated the Government's commitment to reforming the model of health-care delivery so that more and better quality care is delivered in the community.[323] A special allocation of €35 million for mental health was provided in Budget 2012 in line with the Programme for Government commitments. Funding from this special allocation is to be used primarily to strengthen CMHTs in both adult and children's mental health services. The Minister also stated that high standards in services, facilities and inpatient care must be the norm without exception and mental health services must be recovery-oriented and put service users, their families and carers at the centre of care.

In 2007 the Mental Health Commission published a *Quality Framework for Mental Health Services in Ireland*.[324] The framework is based on eight themes, underpinned by 24 standards and 163 criteria. A toolkit has been developed to accompany the framework. The themes are:

- Provision of a holistic seamless service and the full continuum of care provided by a multidisciplinary team
- Respectful, empathetic relationships between people using the mental health services and those providing them

- An empowering approach to service delivery that is beneficial to people using the service and those providing it
- A quality physical environment that promotes good health and upholds the security and safety of service users
- Access to services
- Family/chosen advocate involvement and support
- Staff skills, expertise and morale, which are key influences in the delivery of a quality mental health service
- Systematic evaluation and review of mental health services underpinned by best practice, which will enable providers to deliver quality services

In May 2012 an important national research study, *My World Survey: National Study of Youth Mental Health in Ireland*, was published.[325] The study was a Government-backed research exercise conducted jointly by the UCD School of Psychology and Headstrong – the National Centre for Youth Mental Health. This is the most comprehensive study of the mental health of young people ever conducted in Ireland. The target groups for the My World Survey (MWS) included young people still in second-level education (MWS-SL) and post-second-level education (MWS-PSL). A total of 72 second-level schools randomly selected from the Department of Education and Skills' database participated in the MWS-SL. A total of 6,085 adolescents completed the MWS-SL in the age range 12–19 years (median = 14.93 years). Of these, 51 per cent were females. All school years were represented in the study. Participants in the MWS-PSL were drawn from four sample groups: (1) young adults in third-level education, (2) those enrolled on national training courses/schemes, (3) those who were unemployed and (4) those who were employed. A total of 8,221 young adults participated in the MWS-PSL in the age range 17–25 years (median = 20.35 years). Of these, 65 per cent were females. The survey covered second-level educational institutions in each of the 26 counties of Ireland and every university in Ireland. The total sample size was nearly 15,000.

The report quotes separate research that indicates that about 70 per cent of health problems and most mortality among the young arise as a result of mental health difficulties and substance-use disorders[326] and almost 75 per cent of all serious mental health difficulties first emerge between the ages of 15 and 25.[327]

Among the key findings of the report, it was found that the majority of young people were functioning well across a variety of mental health indicators. Across the age span of 12–25, it was evident that mental health difficulties emerged in early adolescence and peaked in the late teens and early 20s. This peak, in general, was coupled with a decrease in protective factors such as self-esteem, optimism and positive coping strategies. This stage in a young person's life, therefore, is a particularly vulnerable period. Gender was seen to be both a risk and a protective factor. For example, males consistently reported higher levels of self-esteem and satisfaction with life compared to females, but they also engaged in more risk-taking behaviour, including problem drinking, substance misuse and violence towards others. Females reported higher levels of perceived social support and help-seeking behaviours but also engaged in more avoidant coping strategies compared to males.

In order to broaden the understanding of being a young person in Ireland today, the data was analysed not just descriptively but also across a number of key themes. The following themes were found to be significantly related to key mental health indicators, as measured by the MWS:

- 'One good adult' is important in the mental well-being of young people.
- Excessive drinking has very negative consequences for the mental health and adjustment of young people.
- Young adults' experiences of financial stress are strongly related to their mental health and well-being.
- Rates of suicidal thoughts, self-harm and suicide attempts were found to be higher in young adults who did not seek help or talk about their problems.
- Talking about problems is associated with lower mental health distress and higher positive adjustment.

Based on the data from the emergent themes, the MWS indicates that by asking a young person a number of key screening questions it may be possible to determine their mental health status. These questions have been collated into the MWS At-Risk Index. The MWS brings into focus and highlights the needs of a significant number of young people who are not coping with their lives, and strongly reaffirms the importance of early intervention.

Intellectual Disability

The age, health needs and location of those with intellectual disabilities (ID) provide the context of care delivery for intellectual disability nurses. As those with an ID are living longer, their health needs are increasing. ID policy is promoting the importance of community integration and enabling people with an ID to live as equal and valued members of their communities.

The Health Research Board (HRB) manages two national service-planning databases for people with disabilities on behalf of the Department of Health: the National Intellectual Disability Database (NIDD),[328] established in 1995, and the National Physical and Sensory Disability Database (NPSDD), established in 2002. These databases inform decision-making in relation to the planning of specialised health and personal social services for people with intellectual, physical or sensory disabilities.

According to the HRB's 2010 report, in December 2010 there were 26,484 people registered on the NIDD, representing a prevalence rate of 6.25 per 1,000 of the population. The prevalence rate for mild intellectual disability was 2.09 per 1,000 and the prevalence rate for moderate, severe and profound intellectual disability was 3.69 per 1,000. The prevalence rate among the 0–4-years age group continues to decline, but there has been an overall increase in prevalence in the 55-years-and-over age group. The total number with moderate, severe or profound intellectual disabilities has increased by 39 per cent since the first census of mental handicap in the Republic of Ireland was carried out in 1974 and reflects an increase in the lifespan of people with intellectual disabilities. This changing age profile observed in the data over the past three decades has implications for service planning and service delivery.[329]

The National Disability Strategy was launched in September 2004. It provides for a framework of new supports for people with disabilities and builds on a strong equality framework. It puts the policy of mainstreaming of public services for people with disabilities, which was adopted by the Government in 2000, on a legal footing. The main elements of the strategy are the Disability Act 2005, the Education for Persons with Special Educational Needs Act 2004 and six outline sectoral plans published by government departments.

The Disability Act 2005 defines 'disability' as a substantial restriction in the capacity of the person to carry on a profession, business or occupation in the State or to participate in social or cultural life in the State by reason of an enduring physical, sensory, mental health or intellectual impairment. Part 2 of the Act provides a statute-based right for people with disabilities to an assessment of disability-related health, personal social service and education needs.

The *National Disability Strategy Towards 2016: Strategic Document*[330] sets a number of high-level, long-term objectives for people with disabilities: every person with a disability would have access to an income which is sufficient to sustain an acceptable standard of living; every person with a disability would, consistent with their needs and abilities, have access to appropriate health, education, employment and training and personal social services; every person with a disability would have access to public spaces, buildings, transport, information, advocacy and other public services and appropriate housing; every person with a disability would be supported to enable them, as far as possible, to lead full and independent lives, to participate in work and society and to maximise their potential; and carers would be acknowledged and supported in their caring role.

The majority of intellectual disability service provision occurs in settings that cater for groups of people separate from the rest of the community.[331] Most day service occurs in segregated group settings (approximately 90 per cent) and most residential services are provided in segregated group settings (approximately 90 per cent). Many of the individuals in disability services receive what are sometimes described as 'wraparound' services from a single provider. This means the person receives a residential service (i.e. a place to live and daily supports), a day service (i.e. occupation of varying types up to five days a week) and also a variety of health services and other personal social services, depending on their needs. These are all currently funded by the disability services programme budget through the health vote.

In July 2012 the Department of Health published a value for money review of the disability services programme entitled *Value for Money and Policy Review of Disability Services in Ireland*.[332] The purpose of the review was to assess how well current services for people with disabilities meet their objectives and support the future planning and development of services, and to make recommendations that will ensure that the very substantial funding provided to the sector is used to maximum benefit for persons with disabilities, having regard to overall resource constraints which affect all sectors at this time. The review was made up of two strands: an examination of the effectiveness and efficiency of the current disability services programme, and a review of current policy in relation to Department of Health funded disability services. The review proposes a fundamental change in approach to the governance, funding and focus of the disability services programme, with the migration from an approach that is predominantly centred on group-based service delivery towards a model of person-centred and individually chosen supports. The recommended model of supports should be underpinned by a more effective method of assessing need, allocating resources and monitoring resource use. A re-articulated vision and goals are proposed, with a recommendation that a set of realistic, meaningful and quantifiable objectives be developed to support their realisation. The achievement of measurable outcomes and quality for service users at the most economically viable cost underpins the recommendations.

In 2011 the HSE published *Time to Move on from Congregated Settings: A Strategy for Community Inclusion*.[333] According to the strategy, public policy in Ireland over the past twenty years has favoured the development of community-based services. *Needs and Abilities*,[334] the policy for people with intellectual disabilities, published in 1990, made detailed recommendations for discontinuing residential provision that was not domestic in scale. It proposed a range of community-based alternatives, including forms of adult foster care and supports for families to enable them to maintain their family member in a home situation. In 1996 the Review Group on Health and Personal Social Services for People with Physical and Sensory Disabilities' *Towards an Independent Future*[335] also signalled a move away from large institutions, towards small living units and mainstream housing provision. At that time, too, *A Strategy for Equality: Report of the Commission on the Status of People with Disabilities*[336] laid the foundation for the National Disability Strategy in 2004.[337] The strategy gives effect to the Government's mainstreaming policy, which includes the mainstreaming of housing provision for people with disabilities. In response to public policy and investment, the numbers in the congregated settings have been declining and most centres have made arrangements to enable residents to move into the community. However, admissions have continued and, over the period 1999–2008, were marginally higher than numbers leaving the congregated settings.[338]

In spite of the advances made in moving people from institutional to community-based settings, 4,000 adults with disabilities continue to reside and live out their lives in large congregated settings.[339] Accommodating people in these settings clearly runs counter to the State policy of inclusion and full citizenship. In 2007 the HSE set up a working group on congregated settings to develop a national plan and change programme for transferring this group of people to the community. The working group had the following terms of reference and objectives:

- To identify the number of congregated settings and the numbers of people currently living in these settings
- To develop a comprehensive profile of the client group in each setting, in terms of numbers, age, nature of disability and support needs
- To identify the costs of the current service provision
- To estimate the range of services required in order to provide alternative living arrangements
- To develop a framework based on best international practice and up-to-date research to guide the transfer of identified individuals from congregated settings to a community-based setting
- To develop a national plan and change programme for transferring people to the community
- To indicate the likely capital and revenue costs of implementing the programme, with particular reference to an assessment of resources, including capital that can be redeployed/reallocated
- To detail a communication strategy to disseminate the framework for the project and the proposed implementation plan

The working group defined congregated settings as settings where ten or more people with disabilities were living. The report of the working group, *Time to Move on from Congregated Settings: A Strategy for Community Inclusion*,[340] proposed a new model of support in the community, which envisaged that people living in congregated settings would move to dispersed forms of housing in ordinary communities provided mainly by housing authorities. These people would have the same entitlement to mainstream community health and social services as any other citizen, such as GP services, home help and public health nursing services, and access to primary care teams. They would also have access to specialised services and hospital services based on an individual assessment. They would get the supports they needed to help them to live independently and to be part of their local community. A core value underpinning the proposal was that people would make their own life choices; neither the HSE nor service providers own a client but have a responsibility to maximise their independence.[341]

The report stated that the supports provided for people with disabilities must be driven by values of equality, the right of individuals to be part of their community, to plan for their own lives and make their own choices and to get the personal supports they need for their independence. Such expectations should be underpinned by legislation and policy. Person-centred planning should be tailored to individual needs, wishes and choices.

In July 2012 a national implementation framework to support the Government's national housing strategy for people with a disability was published.[342] The implementation framework was developed by an implementation planning group chaired by the Department of the Environment, Community and Local Government, in conjunction with the Department of Health and representatives from the HSE, the Department of Public Expenditure and Reform, the City and County Managers' Association and the Housing Agency. The implementation framework sets out a range of priority actions to support people with disabilities to live in communities as independently as possible, by providing mainstream assessment of housing needs and appropriate housing solutions. The implementation framework is intended to support the Government's commitment to move almost 5,000 people with intellectual, physical and mental health disabilities from institutions to community living over the next seven years.

The health needs of people with an ID are greater and more complex than, and often present differently from, those of the general population.[343] Specific conditions are associated with people with an ID and require additional consideration by service providers.[344] The UK National Health Service's (NHS) 'Health Needs Annual Evidence Update 2010'[345] focused on five key themes relating to the health needs of people with learning/intellectual disabilities: cancer, coronary heart disease, challenging behaviour, epilepsy and respiratory illness. The healthcare needs of people with learning disabilities are well documented in the literature.[346] Health needs might be related to disabilities (e.g. epilepsy and sensory deficits), syndrome-related (e.g. hypothyroidism in people with Down syndrome) or secondary to them (e.g. obesity and reflux disease). People with an intellectual disability also visit primary care professionals less often than would be expected; they receive fewer screening tests and fewer health investigations despite evidence that regular and repeated health checking in primary care can identify previously unrecognised healthcare needs.[347] Furthermore, people with an ID are more likely to have communication impairments that affect their own and others' ability to recognise any deterioration in health status and contribute to inequalities in their healthcare.[348] In tandem with the increasing evidence emerging internationally around the health needs of people with an intellectual disability, many ID services are aiming to provide a social model of service for their clients.

The report *Growing Older with an Intellectual Disability in Ireland 2011* (IDS-TILDA)[349] is a national representative study of 753 people aged 40 and over with an intellectual disability. The results of the study give a profile of people with an ID that is sometimes surprising. For example, the study shows that people with an ID enjoy life more as they get older. Most had a hobby, went on holidays or day trips, engaged in regular leisure pursuits and had social contacts with others. However, they seldom engaged in social activities with friends outside the home and families had limited roles in their lives. Over three-quarters of adults with an ID reported that they never wrote, texted, emailed or used social media tools such as Facebook to contact their family or friends. Moreover, less than 60 per cent used the telephone to make such contacts. Adults with an ID were less likely to own a mobile phone than other adults in the Irish population. The study also found that adults with an ID in Ireland were not actively engaged with their communities and that community 'presence' was not actually equated with 'living' in the community.

Many of the adults in the IDS-TILDA sample, particularly those in the younger age cohorts, reported experiencing good health but there were significant concerns in terms of cardiac issues (including risk factors), epilepsy, constipation, arthritis, osteoporosis, urinary incontinence, falls, cancer and thyroid disease. Younger adults with an ID had a much higher incidence of disease and identifiable risk factors for conditions such as coronary artery disease and stroke than same-age and older cohorts in the general population. Women with an ID had higher risks for many diseases. Sixty-one per cent of

Irish adults with an ID were found to be overweight or obese and the prevalence of diabetes in those aged 50–64 years was double that found for the general population. Women within the mild to moderate range of ID were at the greatest risk.

The study also identified a prevalence of depressive symptomatology among women. It also increased with age, level of ID, sensory loss, reported experience of loneliness and living in a residential centre. Of those who reported a mental ill health diagnosis, over 90 per cent were in receipt of psychiatric support. The prevalence of mental health and emotional problems is greater among persons with an ID than in the general population. Almost one-fifth (18.5 per cent) of Irish adults with an ID reported that they had previously received a diagnosis of depression; this was considerably higher than the 5 per cent reported in the general population. Persons with an ID were at least at the same risk of dementia symptoms as they grew older as the general population, with the risk higher for people with Down syndrome.

Children

RCNs in Ireland will be working in a much more sophisticated and interconnected healthcare policy environment. The new model of paediatric care will drive the context of practice for children's nurses into the future. Children's nurses will provide more complex acute care within the national tertiary centre. The changing model of care delivery will require children's nurses to be prepared to work outside of hospital settings to a greater extent. Skills and competencies for delivery of community care will be important.

In 2000 the Department of Health and Children launched the first comprehensive strategy on children's issues. The National Children's Strategy[350] was a ten-year plan with a vision of an Ireland where children were respected as young citizens with a valued contribution to make and a voice of their own, where all children were cherished and supported by family and the wider society, where they would enjoy a fulfilling childhood and realise their potential. It identified three national goals:

1. Children would have a voice in matters which affected them and their views would be given due weight in accordance with their age and maturity.

2. Children's lives would be better understood and their lives would benefit from evaluation, research and information on their needs, rights and the effectiveness of services.
3. Children would receive quality supports and services to promote all aspects of their development.

These aspirations and ideals were articulated during a period when the scale of child sexual abuse in Ireland was only beginning to emerge in all of its tragic dimensions.

In 2009 there were 1,107,034 children aged under eighteen living in Ireland. This was almost one-quarter (24.8 per cent) of the total population.[351] In 2010 the Department of Health and Children published *State of the Nation's Children: Ireland 2010*.[352] This report was the third in a biennial series prepared by the Office of the Minister for Children and Youth Affairs (OMCYA) in association with the CSO and the Health Promotion Research Centre at NUIG. It fulfilled a commitment in the National Children's Strategy to publish key indicators of child well-being on a regular basis. The report presented the most current and most reliable administrative, survey and census data on the socio-demographic and child well-being indicators that had been selected to be part of the national data set of child well-being indicators in 2005.

The report gives an interesting profile of the well-being of children in Ireland in 2010:

- Ireland continues to have the highest proportion of children in the EU.
- The majority of child deaths occur in the period of infancy (less than one year of age).
- More than half of the total hospital discharges among children were children under five years of age.
- In 2009 there was a total of 145,749 hospital discharges among children.
- The most common reported principal diagnosis recorded was 'diseases of the respiratory system' (13.0 per cent), followed by 'injury, poisoning and certain other consequences of external causes' (9.7 per cent).
- Other diagnoses included diseases of the digestive system, congenital malformations, chromosomal abnormalities and neoplasms.

- The numbers of hospital discharges among children with a diagnosis of 'transport accidents', 'intentional self-harm' and 'accidental poisoning' continue to fall.
- Almost one-quarter of seven-year-old children are either over-weight or obese.
- Approximately six in ten children registered as having an intellectual disability are boys.
- Approximately one in four children on the national physical and sensory disability database are registered as having multiple disabilities.
- The number of cases of confirmed child abuse has increased.
- Children in Ireland have the highest levels of physical activity among 41 OECD countries.
- There has been an increase in the number of children admitted to psychiatric hospitals.

In June 2011 the Government established a Department of Children and Youth Affairs and appointed a Minister for Children with responsibility for the Department. The Department was as a result of a Government decision to consolidate a range of functions that were previously the responsibilities of the Minister for Health, the Minister for Education and Skills, the Minister for Justice and Law Reform and the Minister for Community, Rural and Gaeltacht Affairs. It brings together a number of key areas of policy and provision for children and young people, including OMCYA, the National Educational Welfare Board (NEWB), the Family Support Agency (FSA) and, from January 2012, the detention schools operated by the Irish Youth Justice Service (IYJS). Two important organisations are also included in the overall structure: the Adoption Authority of Ireland and the Office of the Ombudsman for Children.

The Department has a key leadership role in promoting integration at the level of policy and service delivery. It will focus on harmonising policy issues that affect children in areas such as early childhood care and education, youth justice, child welfare and protection, children and young people's participation, research on children and young people, youth work and cross-cutting initiatives for children.

In November 2011 the Department published the *National Strategy for Research and Data on Children's Lives 2011–2016*.[353] The strategy seeks to coordinate and mobilise research and data across a range of bodies in order to achieve a better understanding of children's lives. It is of relevance to a wide variety of stakeholders. The strategy sets an action plan under five key objectives, expressed as five outcome areas of children's lives, which are based on the national service outcomes defined in *The Agenda for Children's Services: A Policy Handbook.*[354] The five outcomes are that children will be:

- Healthy, both physically and mentally
- Supported in active learning
- Safe from accidental and intentional harm, and secure in the immediate and wider physical environment
- Economically secure
- Part of positive networks of family, friends, neighbours and community, and included and participating in society

The strategy also identified four key issues that cut across research and data needs in all areas of children's lives:

- Development of a national strategic approach to information around children's lives
- Improvement of administrative data systems
- Building capacity across all areas of research and data development, particularly analytic capability
- Supporting evidence-informed policy and practice

In 2012 the Department published the *Report of the Independent Child Death Review Group 2000–2010,*[355] which had been commissioned to look into the deaths of children in care or known to the HSE. The report identified a number of systematic failures in the services in relation to the 196 deaths that were reviewed. These included poor risk assessment, poor coordination between services and poor flow of information. It also identified that there was limited access to specialist assessment and therapeutic services, limited inter-agency cooperation for children and families with complex needs and a lack of early intervention. The report made a number of important recommendations in relation to the provision of services for children in care or known to the services. These included:

1. A child death review unit should be established within the Department of Children and Youth Affairs (although other models, including its incorporation in the Office of the

Ombudsman for Children, are also possible). The unit would automatically have the right to investigate the death of any young person who is in the care of the HSE, in aftercare or known to the HSE. It should publish an annual review to the Oireachtas.

2. The operation of the in camera rule must be addressed to allow for transparency and accountability in child care cases. Information gathered in such proceedings must be subject to review and reporting, while at all times protecting the identity of the child and family members.

3. There must be a free flow of information shared between agencies involved in child protection services so as to ensure consistency in the level of protection provided to vulnerable children.

4. A root-and-branch reform of child protection services must be carried out. Each and every person must take responsibility for his/her role in promoting the welfare of children and ensuring their protection.

5. Thorough and comprehensive audits must be conducted of the systems and procedures operating in the child protection system.

6. The report found many of the concerns raised in the report had arisen from 'systematic failures'. It cited a number of 'logical steps' that needed to be followed, factors that were not overly complicated. These included:

   i. risk and mental health assessments of each child
   ii. intervention at the earliest stage where warranted
   iii. regular and clear communication between the HSE and families
   iv. seeking of assistance from courts where necessary
   v. assignment of a social worker to a child and avoidance of constant changing of social workers
   vi. identification of appropriate placements for a child
   vii. identification of necessary services to meet a child's needs, followed by prompt referral to those services
   viii. regular care reviews
   ix. adequate professional supervision and support
   x. completion of critical incident reports when required
   xi. keeping of proper records
   xii. provision of adequate support for foster families
   xiii. provision of adequate aftercare

The Minister for Children and Youth Affairs welcomed the recommendations of the report[356] and indicated that HIQA would assume a new role in relation to the oversight of child protection services[357] and that provisions would be made for the implementation of the recommendation that there should be an independent child death review unit.

The Programme for Government 2011[358] has a number of commitments to children, including a referendum (subsequently held and approved) to amend the Constitution to ensure that children's rights are strengthened, construction of the new National Children's Hospital and a new area-based approach to child poverty.

The National Paediatric Hospital Development Board has published a 'National Model of Care for Paediatric Healthcare in Ireland'.[359] As part of this model, the new National Children's Hospital will be a central component of an integrated healthcare system for Ireland's children, young people and their families. This system will be based on a national network of interconnected elements from GPs and local health centres, through local and regional hospitals, right up to one national tertiary hospital, the new National Children's Hospital. The network will require standardised processes and protocols that apply at all levels of the network so that children and young people receive the highest standard of care relative to their clinical needs irrespective of where they enter the network.

This new national model is built on a number of fundamental principles: care will be provided as close to the child's or young person's home as possible, depending on their clinical needs; care will be provided within the network at the appropriate level, in order to use resources efficiently; where clinically appropriate, short-stay or ambulatory day care will be provided in preference to inpatient care; and parents and family will be supported to engage with and contribute to the care, treatment and healing process.

The new National Children's Hospital will have 445 beds (392 inpatient beds and 53 day-care beds) to meet paediatric healthcare demands projected to peak in 2030.[360] The configuration of these beds conforms to international best-practice trends, resulting in a higher proportion of both critical care and day-care beds. The critical care units will include cardiac and neurosurgical critical care beds, paediatric and neonatal intensive care, and high dependency beds catering for newborn babies requiring specialist intervention. Dedicated facilities are also planned for long-term ventilated children, who no longer need critical care accommodation. Access to paediatric and neonatal critical care services will be supported by a centralised national transport and retrieval service, with helipad access, based at the hospital. Within the inpatient bed configuration, a specific allocation will be made for '23-hour beds' to accommodate an overnight stay following specific elective procedures and interventions, as well as an allocation of 'acute assessment beds' for direct admissions from the ED and urgent care centre.

In November 2012 the Government decided that the new National Children's Hospital would be located at the St James's Hospital campus in Dublin.

An important part of the Programme for Government that referred to the needs of children was the commitment to hold a referendum to strengthen the protection of children in the Constitution. The Programme for Government stated that the wording of the referendum would be along the lines of that proposed by the All Party Oireachtas Joint Committee on the Constitutional Amendment on Children.[361] The referendum was held on 10 November 2012 and the Amendment was approved. The principles of the constitutional change include:

- A general recognition and affirmation of the rights of children
- Provision for the State in certain cases to intervene to protect a child where their parents fail to do so
- Provision to ensure that the law treats all children equally in law, whether or not their parents are married, including in relation to the law on adoption
- Provision to enable a requirement that the best interests of children be regarded as the paramount consideration in the resolution of proceedings affecting children
- Provision to enable a requirement that the views of children be ascertained and given due weight according to their age and maturity in proceedings affecting children

Care of the Elderly

According to the WHO, most developed world countries have accepted the chronological age of 65 years as a definition of an 'elderly' or 'older' person.[362] In Ireland, there are many thousands of nurses who dedicate their working lives to the care of older people. Recent publications and reports on this important area of care (e.g. from An Bord Altranais and HIQA) have tended to use the term

Table 14: Growth in Elderly Population in Ireland, 2002–2036

Age	Actuals				Projected			
	2002	2006	2011	2016	2021	2026	2031	2036
>65 <70	133,474	144,447	175,002	213,004	231,654	257,448	283,886	307,662
>70 <75	112,129	118,320	131,839	161,331	198,129	217,552	243,812	270,742
>75 <80	89,815	92,234	99,953	113,375	141,231	175,892	195,818	222,174
>80 <85	58,857	63,746	67,972	75,582	87,943	112,414	142,688	162,030
>85 <90	29,629	32,489	37,482	41,577	47,897	57,711	76,423	99,572
>90 <95	9,871	11,754	13,949	17,007	19,864	23,985	30,246	41,957
>95 <99	1,784	2,185	3,001	3,911	5,094	6,321	8,110	10,805
>99	442	462	672	991	1,466	2,107	2,893	4,090
Total	436,001	465,637	529,870	626,778	733,278	853,430	983,876	1,119,032
Total Population	3,917,203	4,163,860	4,416,488	4,601,292	4,735,960	4,837,958	4,916,983	4,982,771
%>65	11%	11%	12%	14%	15%	18%	20%	22%

'care of older persons' in preference to 'care of the elderly'. On the other hand, the national clinical programme refers to 'care of the elderly'. In this book I have used the two expressions interchangeably. I believe there is a value in the use of 'care of the elderly', as it evokes images of a world in which the elders are respected and honoured for their maturity, dignity, experience and wisdom and are a treasured part of our society.

As we outlined in Chapter 2, Ireland has experienced a significant growth in the population of those aged over 65. Table 14[363] illustrates clearly that this group is projected to exceed one million by the year 2036, representing approximately 22 per cent of the population. This would represent an increase of almost 100 per cent on the 2011 figure. The largest growth is projected to happen in those aged over 85: the figures in Table 14 suggest that this group will increase by almost three times.

In 2012 the CSO published a thematic report on the elderly as part of its survey on income and living conditions series.[364] This report updates the *Thematic Report on the Elderly, 2004 and 2009* with 2010 data. It focuses on the income of the elderly (i.e. those aged 65 or over) in Ireland in 2004, 2009 and 2010. It includes information on the composition of the elderly cohort, the level and composition of gross weekly equivalised income, the at risk of poverty rate, the consistent poverty rate and levels of enforced deprivation experienced by the elderly in 2004, 2009 and 2010. A summary of the main results is contained in Table 15.

Table 15: Income and Living Conditions of the Elderly in Ireland

	2004	2009	2010
Average gross weekly equalised income	€289.05	€428.86	€403.23
At risk of poverty rate	27.1%	9.6%	9.6%
Deprivation rate	10.0%	9.5%	9.3%
Consistent poverty rate	3.9%	1.1%	0.9%

In 2007 the National Council published a position paper entitled *Clinical Nurse Specialist and Advanced Nurse Practitioner Roles in Older Persons Nursing*.[365] The paper states that older people are and will continue to be the major users of health and social care. For many older people, and particularly the most frail, the level of need can range from continuing care, interspersed with acute episodes that require rapid access to medical treatment, nursing and therapy.[366] When an acute episode occurs, it is about assisting the person back to health as quickly as possible. If full recovery is not possible, the older person requires support to live a full and productive life with a long-term condition. For those with a terminal illness, the aim of care is to ensure a comfortable and dignified death with full support for the person and their family. As the proportion of older persons in the general population increases, there is a need for nurses to develop a range of new technical skills in order to be able to offer short, focused, effective interventions. However, there will also be an increasing need for the more traditional nursing skills, particularly in relation to helping older people stay healthy and in supporting and enabling those with long-term conditions to live positive lives. Gerontological nursing must remain sufficiently wide to embrace new technically focused functions while sustaining and nurturing core fundamental skills and values. Nursing older people is essentially about supporting, educating, enabling, comforting and encouraging people to live fulfilling, healthy lives.[367]

In 2009 An Bord Altranais published *Professional Guidance for Nurses Working with Older People*.[368] The guidance standards were developed for nurses who work with older people in all healthcare settings. They were also intended as a source of information for the older person and his/her family. The guidance standards clarify the nursing care and services to which older people are entitled and which are their right to receive. The standards also provide a basis on which to develop a nursing vision that facilitates role development and articulates an expected level of professional performance.

Also in 2009, HIQA published the *National Quality Standards for Residential Care Settings for Older People in Ireland*.[369] The document states that, with the demise of the traditional extended family, more and more people are moving into residential care settings, such as nursing homes, as they get older. It also states that there is widespread recognition of the need to protect the rights of residents living in residential care settings and of the need for service providers to be supported in providing excellent quality care. The standards were intended to provide a template for the provision of care for the foreseeable future. They were also intended to provide a baseline for those with responsibility for providing care to assess the quality of care planning, to develop strategically appropriate and sustainable resources, and to provide continuity and stability to the lives of those in their care. The standards also provide clear guidelines for residents, their families and/or their representatives on the rights of a resident living in a residential care setting. The document states that every resident should expect to live as full and as independent a life as possible and should be involved in directing, together with the care provider, their own care. HIQA inspectors carry out inspections of premises across the public, private and voluntary sectors to ensure that the standards are being met and that residents are receiving the highest quality care.

Earlier in this chapter we discussed the national clinical programmes.[370] One of these programmes is dedicated to the care of the elderly. The national care of the elderly clinical programme has been established in the HSE Clinical Strategy and Programmes Directorate.[371] The programme aims to reorganise the way older patients are managed in the health service and to roll out nationally a coordinated, multi-disciplinary and patient-focused disease management programme. The principles underlying the design of the programme will be improved quality of care, improved access for patients and cost-effective care. According to the programme's briefing note, the over-65s account for approximately 10 per cent of the population and 50 per cent of acute hospital resources. The management of these patients' journey through the hospital system, therefore, must be standardised and outcomes measured throughout the country. Hospitals are already at various stages in the development of an organised specialist geriatric service and the care of the elderly clinical programme will build on the services already being established.

The objectives of the programme are identified under the headings of quality, access and cost. Under *quality*, the programme aims to improve the management of acutely ill, frail older adults in the acute hospital; to increase independence in the home or reduce inappropriate admission to nursing homes; to reduce the number of falls in older people; and to improve education of the public, medical professionals, allied health professionals and policy decision shapers. Under the heading of *access*, the programme aims to ensure that every patient has quick access to the right care; to integrate acute and community services for the elderly; and to integrate services between the public and private sectors in order to ensure that appropriate services are available for this client group. Under the heading of *cost*, the programme aims to reduce the number of ED attendances, readmissions, hospital bed days and nursing home bed days by reducing delayed discharges; decreasing average length of stay for those aged over 65 years, 75 years and 85 years; reducing the risk of readmission following discharge; decreasing the risk of re-attendance at ED; improving access to funding for home care support services; and reducing the percentage of inappropriate admissions to long-term care.

In 2012 a research review[372] was carried out as part of the research programme of the Dementia Services Information and Development Centre (DSIDC) in TCD and as part of the preparation for the introduction of Ireland's national dementia strategy, to which the Government had committed in its Programme for Government.[373] The research was summarised and presented in a user-friendly format in a guide to future dementia care in Ireland.[374] The guide states that population ageing will inevitably result in an increase in disability and a very significant increase in the incidence of age-related health problems, especially Alzheimer's disease and the related dementias. Increasing age is by far the single strongest risk factor for dementia and a person at the age of 90 runs a 50 per cent higher risk of developing a dementia compared with someone in their 60s. In fact, according to the guide, over the age of 65 the prevalence of dementia nearly doubles every five years. Worldwide an estimated 35 million people have dementia, and in Europe alone about 7 million people are living with dementia. These figures are expected to double every 20 years. There are 42,000 people in Ireland with dementia, which, according to the guide, is a relatively small proportion of the population compared to other countries with a larger elderly population. However, it is projected that the figures in Ireland will increase significantly over the coming years due to our increasingly ageing population. The guide predicts that, by 2041, there will be about 140,000 people with dementia in Ireland. Currently, there is no cure for dementia and people can live a long time after diagnosis. Dementia is a hugely costly public health issue, more costly than coronary heart disease, cancer and stroke combined. According to the guide, a recent World Alzheimer Report estimated that the global cost of dementia was in the region of US$604 billion.

In 2012 a number of pilot initiatives were introduced around the country (Kinsale, South Tipperary, Stillorgan, Blackrock and Mayo)[375] aimed at assisting people to live at home. The initiatives were financed jointly by funds from the HSE and a private philanthropist. The pilot projects recognise that in the future the treatment of dementia will become a major issue for the health services in

Ireland and it is unsustainable to pretend that people with the condition could be treated in institutions.

The National Council[376] highlights the role that CNSs and ANPs can play in the development of integrated care of the elderly services. According to the National Council, the role of the CNS and the ANP in a care of older persons setting is distinguished by the scope of practice, the educational preparation required, the levels of clinical decision-making, the level of responsibility and finally the level of autonomy. It is important that healthcare providers identify areas for development of the roles of nurses at the level of CNS and ANP. These will include services provided by CNSs and ANPs which, while not specific to older persons, can ensure that the older person's complex health needs are assessed in an appropriate and timely manner and that referral to acute services, community services or voluntary services is facilitated efficiently. Examples of such posts where CNSs and ANPs already play important roles and where the holders of these posts manage significant caseloads include stroke care, heart failure, chronic disease and emergency care. According to the National Council, there are already significant numbers of CNSs working in general practices in the community and managing caseloads of chronic conditions, such as COPD, that match those seen by the GP. Other areas include the provision of diagnostic tests, management plans and the management of referral pathways for clients and families at all stages of illnesses such as dementia, circulatory diseases, malignant neoplasms and respiratory diseases. Primary care, therefore, is an area where the role of the CNS and ANP could be developed significantly.

One of the greatest challenges in the provision of care for older people relates to the provision of end-of-life and palliative care. In 2008 the Irish Centre for Social Gerontology at the National University of Ireland conducted a study on behalf of the Hospice Friendly Hospitals Programme and the National Council on Ageing and Older People. A report was published entitled *End-of-Life Care for Older People in Acute and Long-Stay Care Settings in Ireland*.[377] The report details the results of research that focuses, for the first time in Ireland, on the quality of life and quality of care at the end of life for older people in various care settings, including acute hospitals, public extended care units, private nursing homes, voluntary nursing homes and welfare homes. The report provides a new model for care at the end of life which goes beyond specialist palliative care provision to embrace a compassionate approach that supports older people who are living with, or dying from, progressive, chronic and life-threatening conditions, and attends to all their needs: physical, psychological, social and spiritual. The report states that the provision of good end-of-life care should be driven primarily by the concern to enhance quality of life at the end of life and should encompass all of its determinants and components. The report also provides a comprehensive account of current legal issues surrounding end-of-life decision-making in Ireland and states that a robust legal framework is required to guarantee autonomy in decision-making, which is important for quality of life at the end of life. The study raises many important issues for policy-makers and for service planners and providers. Most fundamentally, however, it raises the question of the value placed by our society on how its members are supported and cared for at the end of their lives.

In 2011 the WHO published *Palliative Care for Older People: Better Practices*.[378] This publication built on earlier work in 2004 – *The Solid Facts – Palliative Care*[379] and *Better Palliative Care for Older People*.[380] The first publication in the series builds a detailed picture of the comprehensive nature of palliative care, describing key trends and principles and discussing their policy implications. The second publication focused on the special needs of older people and the major public health challenge they represent. It provided evidence that the needs of this vulnerable group are far from being met. Addressing this gap should be a prime public health concern. The 2011 publication builds on the previous two by giving specific examples of promising or better practices in palliative care for older people along with evidence of their effectiveness when this is available. The project was the work of a European Association for Palliative Care Task Force. The study states that older people suffer unnecessarily, owing to widespread under-assessment and under-treatment of their problems and lack of access to palliative care. This WHO report should be considered together with the palliative care study carried out in Ireland by the HSE and the Irish Hospice Foundation discussed earlier in this chapter in the section on chronic diseases. The study *Palliative Care for All: Integrating Palliative Care into Disease Management Frameworks*[381] makes the point that palliative care is relevant not just for end-of-life diseases. It has a very important role to play in the management of all chronic life-limiting diseases regardless of the age of the sufferer.

Carers

In July 2012 the Department of Health published the first strategy ever dedicated to the role of carers in Irish society, *The National Carers' Strategy – Recognised, Supported, Empowered.*[382] The strategy defines a carer as someone who is providing an ongoing significant level of care to a person who is in need of that care in the home due to illness, disability or frailty. The results of Census 2011 published by the CSO[383] show that every day in Ireland, tens of thousands of family members, friends, partners, parents, children and neighbours provide care to someone who, through a variety of circumstances, needs it. These are Ireland's carers and what they do not only makes a profound difference to the health, well-being and quality of life of those they care for, but also makes an important, often unacknowledged, contribution to the economy.

Census 2011 showed that 187,112 people in Ireland identified themselves as carers (4.1 per cent of the population). Of these:

- 80,891 (43 per cent) provide up to two hours of care per day
- 29,255 (16 per cent) provide between two and four hours of care per day
- 39,982 (21 per cent) provide full-time care (i.e. 43 or more hours per week)
- 15,175 (8 per cent) provide care 24 hours a day
- 73,999 (39 per cent) are males and 114,113 (61 per cent) are female
- The number of male carers has increased by 20 per cent since 2006
- The dominant age cohorts in the caring population are 40–49 years and 50–59 years
- 4,244 carers are aged between 15 and 19 years
- 4,228 carers are aged under 15 years
- 1,838 carers are aged under 10 years

In 2010 the CSO published a special report on carers as part of its series of Quarterly National Household Surveys.[384] That survey showed that at that time:

- 64 per cent of carers were women
- 48 per cent of carers were aged 45–64
- 32 per cent of carers worked full-time

- Four in ten carers were the sole carer for the person they looked after
- Half of all carers cared for someone in the same household
- 47 per cent spent more than 15 hours per week providing care; 21 per cent spent more than 57 hours per week
- Four in ten carers look after a parent or parent-in-law
- Overall, 7 per cent of carers were looking after a child aged 15 years or under and over half (53 per cent) were looking after someone aged 75 years and over

The Irish Longitudinal Study on Aging (TILDA)[385] found that 80 per cent of the main caregivers to people over the age of 50 years were themselves aged 50 years and over and approximately one in five of these were aged over 65 years. They were predominantly the spouse of the person being cared for.

The national carer's strategy sets out four national goals for carers:

- Recognise the value and contribution of carers and promote their inclusion in decisions relating to the person they are caring for
- Support carers to manage their physical, mental and emotional health and well-being
- Support carers to care with confidence through the provision of adequate information, training, services and supports
- Empower carers to participate as fully as possible in economic and social life

The strategy recognises that caring may adversely affect a carer's financial situation, particularly if they have to give up work to become a full-time carer or if they have additional expenses associated with caring, such as fuel, special dietary requirements, transport and medical expenses. In recognition of the financial assistance required by some carers, the Carer's Allowance is a means-tested income support for carers who look after people in need of attention on a full-time basis. If a person is providing full-time care to more than one person, the weekly rate payable is increased by 50 per cent. A Half-Rate Carer's Allowance is also available for people in receipt of another social welfare entitlement. Carer's Benefit is a payment for people who have made social insurance contributions, who have recently left the workforce and are looking after somebody in need of full-time care and attention. In March 2012 approximately 50,500 people were in receipt of Carer's Allowance (including the Half-Rate Carer's Allowance). Approximately 22,000 of these receive the Half-Rate Carer's Allowance. In May 2012 1,608 carers were in receipt of Carer's Benefit.

The strategy identifies a number of key actions that need to be taken to achieve the four goals of the strategy and puts in place a monitoring and reporting system that will require periodic reports on progress to be published and presented to the Government.

Delivering an Integrated Service

The Programme for Government 2011 is committed to continued progress towards the development of a fully integrated health service. Integration needs to happen, in the first instance, within the institutions themselves. This will involve the bringing together of complementary areas of activity under a single clinical director. It will also, where appropriate, mean integration between different institutions, involving the integration of smaller units located within the community, or local, regional and national units of service delivery within a particular speciality area. Boundaries of service delivery in institutional and community settings will, therefore, disappear. The emphasis is on the service, not the location of the service, the patient and the care pathway that he or she must travel and not on the administrative or institutional process.[386]

The changes envisaged by this process of integration cannot happen without impacting significantly on the professions. The process of integration extends to the work practices and the divisions that have traditionally kept professionals in silos, answering to one of their own. Service integration requires professional integration, multidisciplinary cooperation and teamwork. This will require a degree of flexibility and teamwork that is not to be found naturally in the health services as they have been traditionally configured. It represents an approach to service delivery that is based on flexible skill mix models, adapted to the needs of the patients. In the case of nursing and midwifery, it will include working with medical consultants, health and social care professionals and healthcare assistants as a matter of course and as part of a continuous team. It will also require of nurses and midwives that they work with the primary care teams and community intervention teams that have begun to emerge within primary care settings.

The challenge for nurses and midwives is particularly considerable because of the scale of their presence within the system and the potential they have to coordinate and pull together the work of others for the benefit of patients. In order to promote a culture of integration across the professions, it will be necessary to consider the opportunities that exist for integrated education and training at both pre-registration and post-registration/CPD levels. Educating, training and learning together on themes and topics of direct interest to the delivery of services can provide a platform for the formation of natural teams in the care setting and promote a culture of integration and cooperation.[387]

CHAPTER 7

Accountability, Clinical Governance and Leadership

The Nurses and Midwives Act 2011[388] places the protection of the public, patient safety and quality of care at the centre of the regulation and development of the professions of nursing and midwifery. The Act contains provisions for regulation of the professions that are characterised by the traits of openness, transparency and accountability. Self-regulation is no more; the professions are now answerable to the public. This reflects what had already happened for other clinical professionals in the Medical Practitioners Act 2007[389] and the Health and Social Care Professionals Act 2005.[390]

As reported in Chapter 2 of this book, in 2012 HIQA published what is likely to become a landmark report on the quality, safety and governance of healthcare in Ireland, which is now referred to as the Tallaght Hospital Report.[391] The report was the outcome of an investigation that was triggered following the death in March 2011 of a patient awaiting admission on a corridor near the emergency department of the hospital. The report contained far-reaching recommendations. Some were local and specific to Tallaght Hospital, but most were national recommendations to be applied across the whole of the health services. The recommendations covered the areas of unscheduled care, scheduled care, board governance, executive management, and planning, accountability and oversight. The Minister for Health described the report as the template for hospital governance that will be the foundation for the governance of the new hospital groups[392] to be established.[393] With the publication of the report, the Minister also announced[394] approval of HIQA's National Standards for Safer Better Care,[395] which had been in draft format until then. As recommended in the report, the Minister announced that he was putting in place, as a priority, an oversight committee to implement the report's recommendations. He also announced that the chief medical officer had referred the report to the Medical Council and An Bord Altranais, asking them to address the significant issues that arose in the report.

During May 2012 the Minister also announced the creation of a new National Office of Clinical Audit (NOCA), which will be located in and run by RCSI.[396] NOCA will design, develop and implement national clinical audit programmes in order to improve patient outcomes and promote patient safety in hospitals. NOCA has been established through the collaboration of the HSE's quality and patient safety directorate and clinical and strategy programmes directorates together with RCSI and the College of Anaesthetists of Ireland. RCSI will be responsible for the administration and operation of NOCA on behalf of the HSE. The inaugural NOCA governance board will comprise members from the HSE, RCSI, the College of Anaesthetists of Ireland, the Irish Institute of Trauma and Orthopaedic Surgery, the Joint Faculty of Intensive Care Medicine of Ireland, the Independent Hospitals Association of Ireland, the HSE's office of nursing and midwifery directorate and public representation. In launching the initiative, the Minister for Health said that clinical audits aim to assess the extent to which care is consistent with best practice. It also assesses the extent to which care achieves expected outcomes. He said that the establishment of NOCA would provide a sustainable governance structure to advance national clinical audits and would bring Ireland in line with international best practice. Clinical audit is a quality-improvement process that seeks to improve patient care and outcomes through systematic review of care against measurable criteria. The establishment of NOCA supports improvements to clinical practice and service delivery in order to benefit the patient. Put simply, this is about making sure that patients are getting the best treatments performed properly.

The first audit stream under development by NOCA is the Irish audit of surgical mortality. This confidential, independent, peer review audit would provide documented, critical analysis of the outcomes of surgical care. It would allow for the detection of system issues and emerging trends and would enable Irish clinicians to benchmark clinical outcomes against international standards. Three additional audit streams have also been identified for 2012: an Irish national orthopaedic register (to record and monitor joint replacement); a national intensive care audit to monitor patient care and outcomes in intensive care); and an average length of stay audit (collation of data from the average length-of-stay element of the elective surgery programme to inform efficient bed usage in hospitals). The orthopaedic register would provide information on the outcomes of joint replacements and identify risk factors. Implant performance and patient outcomes would be recorded in order to provide feedback to surgeons. The national intensive care audit would measure the quality of patient care and levels of activity in intensive care units in order to drive improvements in intensive care units.

The importance of clinical audits had been highlighted in the Report of the Commission on Patient Safety, *Building a Culture of Patient Safety*.[397] As a result of the recommendations contained in this report, the Patient Safety First Initiative[398] was established, a key component of which was the creation of the National Framework for Clinical Effectiveness and the NCEC.[399] The NCEC provides guidance on the development of clinical guidelines to support evidence-based practice and on the use of clinical audits to improve patient care and outcomes.

It is clear, therefore, that protection of the public, patient safety and quality of care represent the core agenda for the health services for the foreseeable future. This is reflected in the way in which the management and control structures within the services are evolving. The emergence of clinical directorates[400] as the preferred way to organise the delivery of health services underlines the importance of clinical accountability and interdisciplinary shared responsibility. The creation by the HSE of the quality and clinical care directorate and the quality and patient safety directorate are also clear indicators of the importance of this agenda. The processes, protocols, guidance and review mechanisms that are being put in place are designed to ensure that services are delivered in a manner that ensures that the challenges set by this core agenda are met.

There are a number of key concepts that are at the heart of this agenda: accountability, clinical governance and leadership.

Accountability

The HSE defines 'accountability'[401] as a situation in which members of staff have a defined responsibility within an organisation and are accountable or answerable for that. 'Accountability' describes the mechanism by which progress and success are recognised, remedial action is initiated or whereby sanctions (warnings, suspension, deregistration, etc.) are imposed. The Tallaght Hospital Report[402] stated that accountability was demonstrated by service providers accepting responsibility for their decisions and behaviours as service providers and for the consequences for service users, families and carers.

In 2010 the quality and clinical care directorate produced a guidance document on what is meant by 'clear accountability arrangements', which it is obliged to put in place under the terms of the Framework for Integrated Quality, Safety and Risk Management.[403] The need for such a framework emerged from the recommendations of *Building a Culture of Patient Safety*[404] and from the Framework for the Corporate and Financial Governance of the Health Service Executive,[405] which sets out the guiding principles on how the HSE should be managed. The guidance document defined the core value for clear accountability as follows: 'We are responsible and accountable for delivering safe, high-quality, cost-effective care that achieves the best possible health and social care outcomes for people in Ireland.'[406] This core value applies at the individual staff level and at the healthcare organisation level.

At the individual level, each member of staff, nurse or midwife, has personal responsibility for being competent in all aspects of their work; recognising and working within the limits of their competence; reviewing and auditing the standards of the care/service they provide; and cooperating fully with external reviews, audits and inquiries. Where an individual is not satisfied with the standards of care/service being provided, or is of the opinion that they do not have the capacity to deliver the care/service to the required standard, they are responsible for taking steps to resolve problems, exploring all options. If that is not sufficient to remedy the problem, they are obliged to draw the matter to the attention of their line manager. The individual member of staff also has responsibility to provide guidance and support to those whom they hold to account to enable them to exercise their responsibility and authority effectively. This should include regular, timely and relevant management information, training and development in the required skills and competencies and confronting any failures in a constructive way.

The guidance document also made it clear that the individual member of staff, nurse or midwife, had personal responsibility to clearly establish the following:

- What they were accountable for (adhering to the standards of care/service expected of them)
- The results they must deliver, and the resources – financial and human – that are allocated to them
- The lines of accountability for their responsibilities (who is their line manager?)
- Any line management responsibilities that they hold for colleagues or staff
- Their personal responsibilities for the quality and standards of care/service provided by teams of which they are a member (this is particularly important in circumstances in which responsibility for providing care/service is spread between a number of practitioners, departments and/or different agencies)
- The responsibilities of others (staff/teams/agencies, etc.) with whom they work and the associated interdependencies (clarity on this issue is vital to achieving seamless delivery of care for the service user)
- The scope and limits of their authority (the types of decisions they may make without reference to their line manager or higher authority)
- The overall parameters within which their decisions must be made (the organisational values, policies, rules and regulations they must abide by, and the behavioural standards to which they will be expected to conform)
- How their results and the exercise of their responsibility and authority will be monitored and assessed

Applied at the level of the organisation, the guidance document states that the core value means that there is openness, transparency and honesty about the mission, organisational structure, decision-making processes and actions of the organisation. This includes the provision of clear information about the respective functions of boards and their executives. It requires the organisation to describe clearly the hierarchy of authority within which they operate and define the single-point accountability at each level of the organisational structure. The organisation must be clear about the responsibilities and liabilities of individuals/committees/ groups within the organisation, paying particular attention to the interdependencies between units where care and responsibilities are coordinated across various personnel, functions, activities and operating units within and outside the organisation. The organisation must also ensure that responsible individuals are vested with the requisite authority and that individuals/committees/groups are held accountable for their responsibilities. According to the guidance document, this also means that at all times during an episode of care there is clarity about who is the responsible clinician accountable for the service user.

The guidance document also states that a prerequisite for the application of the core value at the level of the organisation is active communication with service users about the organisation (including information on access, treatment options, performance information on quality of care and service user safety) and making information about the organisation publicly available. This active communication is also required internally, with staff within the organisation and with other key stakeholders outside the organisation. Active communication includes listening, providing opportunities for comments to be made, taking on board suggestions, provisions for the protection of whistleblowers and providing assurances that service users, staff and other stakeholders will not be negatively affected by raising concerns.

Accountability for the organisation, according to the guidance document, also includes ensuring that there is adequate internal monitoring and review of structures, systems and processes for accountability and that the information generated is used to support continuous quality improvement. This monitoring and review should result in information that permits objective comparison of results against targets and standards. The organisation should also obtain periodic, external, independent assurance on the effectiveness of its structures, systems and processes for accountability and ensure that this information is used to support continuous quality improvement. This assurance will result in information that permits objective comparison of results against targets and standards. Finally, the organisation must also take appropriate action in cases where there have been failings in the delivery of safe, high-quality, cost-effective care, cooperate fully with external reviews, audits and inquiries, and acknowledge the need for sanctions that are both effective and fair.

Accountability is a key factor in ensuring that healthcare professionals focus constantly on the protection of the public, patient safety and quality in the delivery of their services. In order to ensure that accountability is a reality in the working life of all healthcare workers, what is required is a system of clinical governance.

Clinical Governance

Clinical governance is defined by the HSE[407] in its guidance document 'Clinical Governance Development', which carries the tag line 'We are all responsible … and how are we doing?' The document defines clinical governance as a system through which service providers are accountable for continuously improving the quality of their clinical practice and safeguarding high standards of care by creating an environment in which excellence in clinical care will flourish. It is an umbrella term that encompasses a range of activities in which healthcare staff should become involved in order to maintain and improve the quality of care they provide to patients and to ensure full accountability of the system to patients.

The HIQA Tallaght Hospital Report[408] defined clinical governance as a system through which service providers were accountable for continuously improving the quality of their clinical practice and safeguarding high standards of care by creating an environment in which excellence in clinical care will flourish. This included mechanisms for monitoring clinical quality and safety through structured programmes, for example, clinical audit.

Traditionally, clinical governance has been described using seven key pillars: clinical effectiveness and research; audit; risk management; education and training; patient and public involvement; using information and information technology; and staffing and staff management.

Clinical governance[409] also defines the culture, the values, the processes and the procedures that must be put in place in order to achieve sustained quality of care in healthcare organisations. Clinical governance involves moving towards a culture where safe, high-quality patient-centred care is ensured by all those involved in the patient's journey. Clinical governance must be a core concern of the board and CEO of a healthcare organisation.

In order to assist health service providers in making decisions and in making choices between options, ten principles for clinical governance development[410] were developed by an interdisciplinary working group within the HSE and were reviewed for clarity and usefulness by health managers, clinical directors, senior nurses and midwives, health and social care professionals, and patient groups. The principles were also intended for utilisation as a guide for clinical governance development, across the continuum of care, in each of the national clinical programmes. The models of care developed by the national clinical programmes are central to the further development of clinical governance. The principles are as follows:

- **Patient first**: This is based on a partnership of care between patients, families, carers and healthcare providers in achieving safe, easily accessible, timely and high-quality service across the continuum of care.
- **Safety**: Proactive identification and control of risks is utilised to achieve effective, efficient and positive outcomes for patients and staff.
- **Personal responsibility**: This is where staff, patients and the population take personal responsibility for their own and others' health needs, where each employee has a current job description setting out the purpose, responsibilities, accountabilities and standards required in their role.
- **Defined authority**: This is the scope given to staff at each level of the organisation to carry out their responsibilities. The individual's authority to act, the resources available and the boundaries of the role are confirmed by their direct line manger.
- **Clear accountability**: This is a system whereby individuals, functions or committees agree accountability to a single individual.
- **Leadership**: This requires motivating people towards a common goal and driving sustainable change to ensure safe, high-quality delivery of clinical care.
- **Interdisciplinary working**: This entails work processes that respect and support the unique contribution of each staff member in the provision of clinical care. Interdisciplinary working focuses on the interdependence between individuals and groups in delivering services. This requires proactive collaboration between all staff.
- **Supporting performance**: This means managing in a supportive way, in a continuous process, taking account of clinical professionalism and autonomy in the organisational setting;

supporting a director/manager in managing the service and employees, thereby contributing to the capability and capacity of the individual and organisation. Measurement of the patient's experience is central in performance measurement.

- **Open culture**: This is a culture of trust, openness, respect and caring where achievements are recognised. Open discussion of error is embedded in everyday practice and communicated openly to patients. Staff willingly report adverse events, so there can be a focus on learning, research and improvement, and appropriate action is taken where there have been failings in the delivery of care.
- **Continuous quality improvement**: This provides a learning environment with a comprehensive programme of quality improvement programmes.

The guidance document stated that these principles should be used within organisations to measure how the organisation's clinical governance structures and processes operate. The clinical governance processes include quality and performance indicators; learning and sharing information; patient and public community involvement; risk management and patient safety; clinical effectiveness and audit; staffing and staff management; information management; capacity and capability. The structures include the clinical governance committee for the organisation as a whole, consisting of the lead (member of the executive or senior management team) for each process, and the local directorate/department/practice meetings (conforming to the principles and processes of clinical governance). Best practice would indicate that regular reviews of both structures and processes are carried out using the principles as indicators of the standards that must be applied.

As already mentioned, the Tallaght Hospital Report[411] contained a number of recommendations on clinical governance to be implemented at a national level. These give a clear illustration of the kinds of clinical governance systems that are required to be put in place in order to ensure that accountability within the system is a reality. In the area of unscheduled care, the report recommended that all hospitals must have the necessary arrangements in place to ensure that there is a named consultant clinically responsible and accountable for a patient's care at all points in the patient journey and throughout their hospital stay, that all hospitals should have the appropriate implementation and monitoring arrangements in place to ensure that on-call clinical teams are available to see patients in the emergency department, and that the HSE should review the current national position of the expanded roles within nursing and allied health professionals and implement a plan to roll out a more extensive programme of expanded practitioners within the appropriate clinical settings and with the necessary clinical governance arrangements in place nationally and locally.

On scheduled care, the report recommended that all hospitals should have effective arrangements in place to ensure that all patient waiting lists are periodically reviewed by a senior clinical decision-maker to ensure that the clinical priority and urgency for each patient is managed and regularly reviewed, and that arrangements should include two-way communication with the patient and their general practitioner. It also recommended that voice recognition and clinical alert software with a formalised process for critical alerts to GPs for abnormal patient imaging results must be put in place in all hospitals and monitored and evaluated on an ongoing basis. It also recommended that all hospitals should consider, where appropriate, safe mechanisms for implementing nurse-led patient discharge processes, with the appropriate supporting clinical governance arrangements.

Clinical governance is not possible without the existence of a related system of corporate governance. The Tallaght Hospital Report defined corporate governance as the system by which services direct and control their functions in order to achieve organisational objectives, manage their business processes, meet required standards of accountability, integrity and propriety, and relate to external stakeholders. The report made a number of far-reaching recommendations that have significant implications for the governance arrangements, structure, composition and functioning of hospital boards and executive management. It also made a number of significant recommendations related to planning, accountability and oversight. Many of these recommendations have important implications for nursing and midwifery.

On the structure and composition of boards, the report recommended that membership of boards should not exceed twelve persons and that these should be selected and appointed through an independent process established by the State and on the basis of having the necessary skills, experience and competencies required to fulfil the role effectively. The chief executive and other designated executive officers (to include, as a minimum, the equivalent of the director of finance, medical/lead clinical director and director of nursing) should be formally in attendance at the board with combined shared corporate accountability for the effective governance and management of the hospital. This was the first time in Ireland that a formal recommendation had been made regarding the inclusion of the director of nursing at board level. The recommendation mirrored developments in the NHS,[412] where the role of the executive nurse is emerging as a key element in the further development of governance systems. This recommendation was further underpinned by recommending that a clear scheme of delegation of accountability from the board to the chief executive and executive directors should be in place. This should include unambiguous delegated executive accountability and responsibility for the quality and safety of patient care. With regard to the executive management of hospitals, and as part of the establishment of the hospital groups/networks,[413] competent, high-performing chief executives and executive directors (including directors of finance, medical/lead clinical director and director of nursing) with clear delegated accountability should be appointed.

The report recommended that boards should have access to whatever information they need to assist them in monitoring the performance of the hospital. A board should have access to the appropriate information in order to fulfil its role of effectively governing the delivery of high-quality, safe and reliable healthcare. This should include the development of a quality and safety assurance framework with key performance indicators (KPIs) to assure patient safety, patients' experience, access and financial management. Every board should use these KPIs and other quality and safety information to assure itself about the quality and safety of care being provided and publish this information. Allied to the requirement for unambiguous delegated accountability to executive management, these recommendations provided a strong framework for holding to account those who have responsibility for the delivery of quality, safe care to the clients of the health services.

The Tallaght Hospital Report confirmed that developments in nursing and midwifery over the previous ten years, particularly with the introduction of the CNS/CMS and ANP/AMP, have the potential to make a substantial contribution to quality, safe and more efficient care within healthcare settings. As noted above, the investigation underpinning the report was triggered by a tragic incident of a death of a patient waiting on a trolley in a corridor adjacent to the ED. The report stated that international evidence and systematic reviews indicated that suitably qualified and experienced nurse practitioners, when working with clear clinical guidelines, reduced waiting times in the ED, improved continuity of patient care and were cost-effective and safe.[414] The report said that, although funding was in place for a second ANP post, the hospital had, over the previous three years, been unsuccessful in filling this post. However, hospitals of a similar size in Dublin had, over the previous years, enhanced their ED services by increasing their number of ANPs.

At the time of the investigation, the ED service was working well during core hours. However, the role of the ANP, due to internal constraints, had not extended to include the requesting of X-rays. In practice, this meant that patients who had been clinically assessed by the ANP and required an X-ray had to wait until an NCHD signed the request form. The report accepted that this challenge was not specific to the hospital and recommended that, nationally, nurse prescribing of imaging diagnostics be supported and expanded. The authority to prescribe ionising radiation and medicinal products is something that had already been approved and agreed by An Bord Altranais in 2008.[415]

According to the report, outside of core hours the minor injury service was provided by the ED clinical staff, rather than ANPs. As a result, it was reported during the interview conducted as part of the investigation that, when the ED was busy, patients with minor injuries sometimes had to wait for extended periods to be seen and treated. The provision of nurse-led minor injuries services at the hospital, if adequately resourced and structured, would effectively reduce the waiting times for patients with minor injuries, improve patient flow and could lead to a more effective utilisation of clinical staff.

These recommendations pose significant challenges for nursing and midwifery in Ireland. As professions and as individual healthcare providers they will be held to account in a manner that has not happened to date for the quality and safety of the care they provide. Nurses and midwives will also be expected to be capable of providing the leadership that is required within the healthcare system to ensure that the voice of the professions is heard. Structures and systems are now being put in place to ensure that there is a place at the corporate table for their voice to be heard. Provision is being made to ensure that nurses and midwives occupy positions of leadership in the management and delivery of healthcare services in all settings. It will be the responsibility of the leaders of the professions to articulate that voice and it will be the responsibility of each individual nurse and midwife professional to ensure that they contribute to the delivery of the health services in a manner that reflects the leadership role that nursing and midwifery can play in delivering quality, safe and efficient care.

Leadership

The HSE defines[416] 'leadership' as getting people to do things using intrinsic motivation, i.e. internal motivators such as knowing that the organisation (in the person of one's manager) cares about one as a person, a sense of ownership of the work (whether individual or collective), of pride in something well done, of satisfaction in a challenge overcome and of meaning to what one does. Leadership represents a key lever for successful transformation towards integrated service delivery. It influences the performance of all professions and grades in providing services for users. Health services require dispersed and collective forms of leadership, alongside active followership, core management practices and organisational direction.[417]

Nursing and midwifery is the largest cohort of healthcare providers within the system. Their role and functions involve the coordination and management of inputs from many other professionals and healthcare workers. They are, therefore, ideally positioned at a central point within the system to be a source of significant leadership in championing the protection of the public, patient safety and quality of care. In 2010 the National Leadership and Innovation Centre for Nursing and Midwifery was established within the Office for Nursing and Midwifery Services Director in the HSE. The aim of the centre is to work with nurses and midwives in building innovation and leadership skills, knowledge and networks to transform healthcare for patients and the public.[418]

The development of leadership skills in nursing and midwifery is also a significant international priority. The International Council of Nurses (ICN) provides leadership development support through the *Leadership for Change*[419] programme. This programme focuses on enhancing effectiveness in health planning and policy development; leadership and management in nursing and health services; developing quality cost-effective nursing services; preparing future managers and leaders, nurses and non-nurses; sustaining development; contributing within the broader health and management teams; influencing curricula changes; and networking nationally, regionally and internationally.

In Ireland, nursing and midwifery professionals are increasingly playing a central role in the development and implementation of the national clinical programmes. However, until now there has been no requirement for the board of the HSE or of the voluntary hospitals and other key healthcare agencies to include representatives from nursing and midwifery. The role of director of nursing does not always include an automatic role on the board of the hospital or care setting in which they operate. The recommendations of the Tallaght Hospital Report[420] have changed that. In future, the director of nursing will have executive management responsibility and will be required to be present at board meetings to give account of his or her role and to articulate the voice of nursing on questions of patient safety, quality and clinical care.

In August 2011 the Department of Health announced that a number of cost-neutral reforms of the hospital system in Ireland would be introduced, including the establishment of a trust system for hospitals based on an analysis of a similar system in England and elsewhere.[421] The Tallaght Hospital Report recommended that the boards of these trusts of hospital groups and the appointment of the executive management group should be established in line with its recommendations. This means that the executive role of the director of nursing/midwifery will become an important part of the development of these trusts/hospital groups. In this context, it is important that consideration should be given to the way in which the role of the nurse executive has developed within the NHS.

In the United Kingdom, the NHS has provided guidance on governance arrangements for NHS foundation trusts. Foundation trusts are required, as a legal minimum, to have a registered nurse or midwife among their executive directors.[422] In Wales, every local health board should have a nurse director and, in Scotland, a nurse executive director should be a member of all NHS boards and special health boards.[423] However, nurse executive representation at board level is not always a statutory requirement, and there is some evidence that the role is less well established where there is no such requirement. For example, the UK Department of Health 'expects' the boards of each new primary care trust (PCT) and strategic health authority to include a director-level nurse.

The leadership role of the nurse executive was the subject of a recent research exercise commissioned by the King's Fund[424] entitled *From Ward to Board*. The King's Fund has developed a programme of work to support nurse executives and NHS trust boards to 'bring the ward to the board'. It is about turning the spotlight firmly on to reviewing clinical quality, and putting patients and how they experience healthcare at the heart of an organisation's work. It set out to explore the role of nurses on the board and how far they were able to influence boards to increase the level of engagement with clinical quality. The first phase of the programme was based on seven pilot sites across the UK. These pilot sites were chosen for the learning they could contribute about the role of the nurse executive in relation to high-quality, board-level clinical engagement, as well as how to manage patient care and improve the quality of the patient experience.

Lessons learned about the role and capabilities of the nurse executives suggest that they have a key role to play in helping to create the right culture and climate to have open discussions about quality; leading by example and constantly reinforcing the importance of clinical quality to all aspects of the business; stimulating discussion about what types of information boards want and need to know in order to assure quality; presenting, analysing and interpreting hard data and identifying the clinical impact of that data; serving as a conduit of information about the patient experience through the use of soft intelligence and compelling narrative; helping boards to tap into the emotional content of the patient experience; and role-modelling appropriate behaviours around presenting and receiving negative feedback from and about patients.

From Ward to Board also identified a number of key capabilities that are important if nurse executives are to work effectively with boards to secure improvements in clinical quality. Nurse executives need to have excellent communication skills and to be able to talk convincingly about the business of the whole organisation, and not limit their contributions to clinical issues. Nurse executives at the pilot sites, who were observed as having an impact in the boardroom, were able to talk convincingly about the business of the whole trust and how clinical quality fitted into this strategically. Where nurse executives limited their contributions to clinical issues, they were more likely to believe that they were defined primarily by their nursing background and to feel sidelined in the boardroom in comparison to their finance colleagues. Nurse executives also needed to be able to draw on a wide range of capabilities, employing a style, tone and body language that reflect authority, confidence and competence. One of the most important competencies is developing emotional intelligence in order to discuss difficult clinical issues with credibility. Nurse executives need to consider the language used to present the patient experience and to avoid the use of business-oriented metrics that fail to accommodate the emotional content of patients' stories. They need to be able to draw on financial and commercial acumen but also retain their clinical focus and emphasis on the human experience.

One of the most valuable aspects of the nurse executive role is the potential to serve as a conduit of information about the realities of the patient journey and to 'bring the ward to the board'. According to the research, the ability of nurse executives to successfully fulfil this role was, in part, attributable to their use of 'soft intelligence'. Presence on the 'shop floor' and nurturing relationships with nursing staff in wards and departments were key elements of this.

The research also identified the need for the nurse executive to be able to nurture key alliances, both within and outside the boardroom, which would support them to be more confident and authoritative in discussing clinical quality at board level. Nurse executives who enjoyed good support from their chief executive were more confident and more commanding of respect, and more courageous and open in the information they brought to the board. The good relationships and mutual support between nurse executives and their medical director peers had the potential for even greater impact on the quality agenda at board level. The research also found that to be effective nurse executives needed to be supported by robust reporting processes around clinical quality and a boardroom environment that was open and interested in this agenda. Where there was an authoritative nurse executive, the board was usually characterised as having robust reporting processes around clinical quality, or at least a strong focus on the issues.

The Royal College of Nursing,[425] in their *RCN Policy Position: Executive Director of Nursing*, stated that every PCT in England should have an executive director of nursing at board level in order to ensure that the voice of nursing is properly represented within the governance of the NHS. According to the Royal College of Nursing, the value that the executive director of nursing at board level brings means that clinical quality and patient care are central to NHS governance. This supports the strategic culture to enable the delivery of high-quality care throughout organisations. The value that nurses at board level bring means that nurses at all levels in the NHS can be enabled to deliver on quality care, including safety, dignity, care and compassion – the core values of nursing. An executive director of nursing on the board will ensure that quality care is the business of the whole organisation. As the shift from acute to community service provision increases, the importance of nursing requires additional strategic oversight at board level to ensure quality care is provided in the community and in a person's own home. This gives added emphasis to the challenges that the health services in Ireland are facing today and provides a benchmark for the role that nursing and midwifery should play.

If nurses and midwives are to be involved at board level in order to shape and define strategy and priorities that are patient-centred and quality driven, they will need to develop the kind of capabilities and competencies identified in the King's Fund research exercise.[426] These competencies mirror earlier research in this area by Carol Huston,[427] which identified key competencies required to prepare nurse leaders for 2020 and the kind of educational models and management development programmes that will be necessary to assure that these skills are present. According to Huston, the nurse leader of 2020 will require a global perspective or mindset regarding healthcare and professional nursing issues; technology skills which facilitate mobility and portability of relationships, interactions and operational processes; expert decision-making skills rooted in empirical science; the ability to create organisational cultures that permeate quality healthcare and patient/worker safety; understanding and appropriately intervening in political processes; highly developed collaborative and team-building skills; the ability to balance authenticity and performance expectations; and being able to envision and proactively adapt to a healthcare system characterised by rapid change and chaos.

In Ireland the role of the director of nursing in both hospital and community settings will continue to be of great importance as the healthcare reform programme is implemented. The intention of the Government to organise hospitals into groups, potentially with trust status,[428] means that the director of nursing will have a key role to play across institutional boundaries. Of course, job descriptions will vary from one clinical care setting to another and from one discipline or area of speciality to another. The overarching trend, however, is towards a situation where the director of

nursing/midwifery is responsible for the management of nursing/
midwifery, not nurses/midwives. His or her contribution to clinical leadership and clinical governance issues and supporting the
nurse/midwife managers responsible for the operational management of the nursing/midwifery resource is a key part of the role.
He or she will also be responsible for ensuring that there is a well-
articulated nursing voice at the corporate decision-making table,
capable of negotiating budgets for the nursing and midwifery
resource for the corporate structure. He or she will lead in the
integration of services and the development of cooperative, multidisciplinary approaches to service development, with the interests
and safety of the patient at the core.

Resource planning and, in particular, nurse forecasting is an
essential component of the kind of leadership input required from
the executive nurse/director of nursing at corporate level within
the health services. In Ireland this is an underdeveloped function, as
highlighted by the recent RN4CAST – Nurse Forecasting in Europe[429]
project, funded under the Seventh Framework Programme of the
European Commission. The study was carried out by DCU as part of
an international consortium including Belgium, Finland, Germany,
Greece, Poland, Spain, Sweden, Switzerland, the Netherlands and
the UK. The overall objective of the RN4CAST project was to expand
typical forecasting models with factors that take into account how
features of work environments and qualifications of the nursing
workforce impact on nurse and patient outcomes. In doing this, a
survey of 1,406 nurses and 285 patients on selected general medical
and surgical wards in a total of 30 different study hospitals across
the Republic of Ireland was carried out using a number of different
survey tools. The research results highlighted the need for a more
developed approach to workforce planning that takes into account
the changing environment in which healthcare is delivered in
Ireland today. This is an area of corporate planning where nursing
and midwifery leadership at the most senior level is required.

Senior nurses and midwives, other than the executive nurse/
director of nursing, also have a key leadership role to play
within the healthcare system. A comprehensive research exercise
commissioned by the National Council,[430] aimed at evaluating the
effectiveness of the role of ANPs/AMPs and CNSs/CMSs within
the Irish health services, identified a number of clinical and professional leadership activities of specialists and advanced practitioners
that are to be found in those who practise at this level. In the clinical

area, the specialist and advanced practitioner guides and coordinates the activities of the multidisciplinary team, introduces and develops patient/client care services, initiates and changes patient/client care through practice development, changes clinical practice through formal education of the multidisciplinary team, takes responsibility for policy and guideline development and implementation, mentors and coaches the multidisciplinary team in clinical practice, and acts as a positive role model of autonomous clinical decision-making and ongoing professional development. In addition, advanced practitioners and specialists engage in a number of professional leadership activities: developing policy at a national and international level, engaging in education outside the service at a national and international level, and engaging in professional organisations and committees at a national and international level.

Within the clinical directorate structure, one of the key leadership roles for the professions is that of the nurse manager,[431] who is a key member of the clinical directorate management team as described in the clinical director profile included in the consultant contract.[432] He or she is operationally accountable to the clinical director on all matters that refer to the management of the nursing/midwifery resource within the clinical directorate. He or she has a professional relationship with the director of nursing/midwifery in all matters of professional standards, quality and development of nursing services. His or her role, together with that of the business manager, is to support and cooperate with the clinical director in the overall planning and management of the directorate. The nurse manager would be expected to contribute to the process of strategic planning for the directorate in all nursing/midwifery and nursing/midwifery-related matters and lead the development of nursing and midwifery roles at the levels of generalist, specialist and advanced practitioner nurse/midwife in line with service needs. The nurse manager should also support clinical training and continuing professional development for the nursing/midwifery resource within the directorate and cooperate with other senior professional colleagues in the development and implementation of multidisciplinary professional development and training initiatives.

The precise description of the role of the nurse/midwife manager is likely to vary from one care setting and one speciality to another. The overarching theme, however, is one of integrated, multidisciplinary teamwork, reporting to the clinical director and maintaining a professional link on behalf of the nursing/midwifery resource with the director of nursing/midwifery. The nurse/midwife manager is also a senior executive within the directorate, with budget and accountability responsibility delegated from the clinical director. He or she needs to be empowered to take control of the environment for which he or she is responsible and to take decisions about the management of that environment in the interests of quality of care, patient safety and best use of resources available.

In addition to the role of nurse manager, the role of the CNM2/CMM2 will continue to be of central importance within the clinical directorate structure at the front-line of the delivery of clinical services.[433] He or she will be responsible for the management of a unit or ward and will, in the majority of cases, provide the key front-line management needs of nurses and midwives in the care setting. The Commission on Nursing[434] defined the functions of clinical nurse managers/clinical midwife managers as providing professional and clinical leadership, managing staffing and staff development, resource management, and facilitating communication. The CNM2/CMM2 should be empowered by the nurse/midwife manager to fulfil all the key front-line management functions within a unit or ward. In order to do that, he or she will require the provision of appropriate information and training and should be involved in determining the resource needs for the unit. The CNM2/CMM2 is usually supported where necessary by a CNM1/CMM1, who will deputise for the CNM2/CMM2 when necessary and provide additional management support in complex care delivery settings. In occasional circumstances (e.g. in large accident and emergency department or large surgical/operating units within large acute hospitals), there may also be the need for a CNM3/CMM3 to provide departmental management cover. The determination of the precise combination of grades required for a particular care setting is a matter for service planning at a local level with the clinical directorate.

The backbone of care delivery within the health services will continue to be provided by the tens of thousands of nurses and midwives who operate at the front-line in acute and primary care settings. The level of practice at which individual nurses or midwives act will depend on where they are in the clinical career pathway, i.e. at generalist, specialist or advanced practice level.

As part of their role within the primary–acute care continuum, nurses and midwives will continue to develop nurse-/midwife-led clinical services. These services should be developed in consultation with the clinical director and other health service managers and should reflect the levels of practice of the individual nurse or midwife. They should include, as appropriate,[435] management of caseloads in both acute and community settings in accordance with agreed practice protocols and in line with their levels of practice; management of early discharge from acute settings and follow-up with the patient/client in the community, including, where appropriate, in their own home; diagnosis of conditions in accordance with agreed practice protocols; treating and prescribing in accordance with agreed practice protocols; referring clients/patients to other areas of service delivery and other professionals in accordance with the needs of the patient/client; taking referrals from other areas of the services and from other professionals in accordance with the needs of the patient/client; and education and empowerment of patients/clients in the community settings and in their own homes in the management of their own health.

Nurses and midwives will prescribe medications in accordance with the provisions of legislation and after having completed the required education and training programmes and having achieved registration as a registered nurse prescriber with An Bord Altranais. Nurses and midwives will incorporate the roles of healthcare assistants, home helps and other support staff into the delivery of their services, as appropriate, in both acute and primary care services, and in line with agreed protocols and practice. They should also continue to develop relationships with medical consultants, doctors and other healthcare professionals in a way that reflects the development of their roles within their career pathways and in line with service needs. This should include identification of complementarity, development of an understanding of what each professional can bring to a multidisciplinary team, breaking down silos of practice, and encouraging a culture of common decision-making, collaborative working and multidisciplinary service delivery.[436]

The *Report of the Commission on Nursing*[437] identified a number of perceptions that relate directly to management and leadership within the professions. In particular, the report pointed to a need for greater internal communication within organisations and highlighted the fact that nurses and midwives, and nursing and midwifery, were not sufficiently involved in strategic planning or in policy and strategy development. This was reflected in a lack of partnership and consultation between general management and nursing and midwifery management and between nursing/midwifery management and nurses/midwives in setting and attaining corporate goals. The report criticised nursing and midwifery management, indicating that it was too preoccupied with hierarchies and the detailed control of nurses and midwives rather than the management of the nursing and midwifery functions.

The report saw a need to examine the recruitment, selection and training of nurse/midwife managers so that the professions would have an effective cohort of leaders capable of responding to changing service needs. It also advocated greater devolution of authority within nursing and midwifery management structures. These issues were also mentioned in a supplementary report prepared for the Commission on Nursing: *Management in the Health Services: The Role of the Nurse.*[438] Responding to this, the Commission made specific recommendations regarding internal communications within health service organisations, professional and personal career planning and the involvement of nurses and midwives in the strategic planning of the nursing and midwifery services. It also made recommendations regarding the roles of nurses and midwives in the management of their professions and their involvement in general management and emphasised leadership in both general management and clinical settings.

The Department of Health and Children subsequently established the institutional structures recommended by the Commission and also set up a high-level steering group on the empowerment of nurses and midwives. In September 2003 the Department issued the final report of the steering group, *Nurses' and Midwives' Understanding and Experiences of Empowerment in Ireland.*[439] This report made reference to an earlier study produced by the OHM,[440] on nursing management competencies, which identified a number of key competencies required for each of the different levels of nursing management. At the top level these should include strategic and system thinking; establishing policy, systems and structures; leading on vision and values; stepping up to the corporate agenda; and adopting a development approach to staff. At middle management level, they should include a proactive approach to planning; effective coordination of resources; an empowering/enabling leadership style; setting and monitoring performance standards; and negotiation skills. At front-line level, they should include planning and organisation of activities and resources; building and leading the team; and leading on clinical practice and service quality. The study also noted a number of generic competencies that should be present throughout nursing and midwifery. These include promoting evidence-based decision-making; building and maintaining relationships; communication and influencing relationships; service initiation and innovation; resilience and composure; integrity and ethical stance; sustained personal commitment and practitioner competence; and professional credibility.

Since the publication of the *Report of the Commission on Nursing*, much progress has been made in the development of leadership for the professions as outlined in this book. In academic institutions, nurses and midwives have attained a status that is equivalent to other healthcare professionals. With the enactment of the Nurses and Midwives Act 2011 and the impending introduction of a new Board, much progress has been made in modernising the regulation of the professions and making them more accountable. At a policy level, there has been progress in ensuring that the voice of the professions is heard. At the clinical level, great strides have been made and nursing and midwifery now occupy a central role in the planning, development and delivery of clinical services. The implementation of the recommendations contained in the Tallaght Hospital Report[441] will ensure that the progress made to date is formally incorporated into the systems and processes of the healthcare system and will provide a place at the centre of the decision-making structures for the voice of nursing and midwifery. In this sense, since the *Report of the Commission on Nursing*, the professions have matured as key partners in the delivery of patient-centred safe care.

In order for nursing and midwifery to fulfil its potential within the healthcare system, nurses and midwives need to engage in further education, training and personal development in areas that are not seen as traditional nursing and midwifery skills. These include strategic planning, finance, economics, IT and a range of communication and negotiation skills required to make an impact at the strategic decision-making levels. Leadership for the professions from the top should ensure that there is coordination and cohesion between all of the elements involved in the healthcare services. This must include regular outreach exercises designed to empower and listen to nurses and midwives at the front-line and to instil in them a vision of the core values of the professions and of their future development within the Irish healthcare services.

CHAPTER 8

Survey of Nursing and Midwifery in the Irish Health Services

In December 2011, as part of the research for this book, I carried out a limited survey of nursing and midwifery, covering some of the key themes in the book. The survey questionnaire is in Appendix 2. The questions in the survey covered topics such as leadership, involvement in planning and development of services, expansion of practice, integration of acute and primary care services, the adequacy of undergraduate and postgraduate education provision, the clinical career pathway, the importance of patient safety, the importance and need for independent regulation of the professions, and the need for accountability and clinical governance in the form of clinical audits, protocols and standards that are focused on identified outcomes and the achievement of key performance indicators.

My intention in conducting the survey was to determine the degree to which key categories of nurses and midwives agree with a number of key positive statements around the themes of this book. The principal target group for the survey was directors of nursing and midwifery and directors of public health nursing. This group accounted for almost 80 per cent of the total sample. The reason for this was my wish to gauge the views of those who have primary responsibility for leading and managing nursing and midwifery in Ireland. The survey also included heads of schools in universities and institutes of technology, directors of CNEs/CMEs and the directors of NMPDUs. A total of 207 questionnaires were distributed by email. The response rate was 34 per cent (see Table 16).

Table 16: Survey Sample

	No.	%
Total questionnaires (sample)	207	100%
Total response	71	34%

The breakdown of the sample categories and the response rate for each category is summarised in Table 17.

Table 17: Sample Categories and Response Rates

Categories	Sample	%	Respondents	%
Directors of nursing, midwifery and public health nursing	164	79%	52	32%
Universities	7	3%	5	71%
Institutes of technology	6	3%	3	50%
CNEs/CMEs	19	9%	4	21%
NMPDUs	11	5%	7	64%
Total	**207**	**100%**	**71**	**34%**

The response rates by categories can be further analysed by amalgamating the clinical/management (all directors of nursing, midwifery and public health nursing), educational (universities and institutes of technology) and development (CNEs/CMEs and NMPDUs) elements. Response rates according to these amalgamated categories are summarised in Table 18.

Table 18: Amalgamated Survey Categories

Categories	Sample	Respondents	%
Clinical/Management	164	52	32%
Education	13	8	62%
Development	30	11	37%
Total	**207**	**71**	**34%**

The limitations of the survey are obvious: it is an informal survey carried out by email; the sample size is small and is not representative of nursing and midwifery as a whole; and it concentrates on the senior management cohort of nursing and midwifery and on the leaders of education and professional development establishments. However, the survey is based on a high-quality and focused list of invitations to respond. The overall response rate (34 per cent) is very satisfactory and the response rate of the largest cohort of invited participants (32 per cent) is also very satisfactory. The survey responses also generated a number of considered unprompted comments, collected in a text box inviting additional comments. These comments provide interesting insights and a more nuanced view of the responses received.

The questions in the survey sought an immediate response to a list of positive statements, offering five possible responses: strongly agree, agree, neutral, disagree and strongly disagree. Respondents were also invited to include comments of their own in a text box at the end of the questionnaire. The results were enlightening.

At the time the survey was in progress, the Nurses and Midwives Act 2011 was still making its way through the legislative process and had not yet been enacted. All of the participants in the survey, however, would have been highly aware of the implications of the Act and would more than likely have been active participants in the consultation process that took place during the previous two years. The question on regulation, therefore, was an important one for the content of this book. The response to this question is illustrated in Figure 2.

Figure 2: Regulation

There is a need for strong, independent regulation of the professions of nursing and midwifery in Ireland, centred on the protection of the public

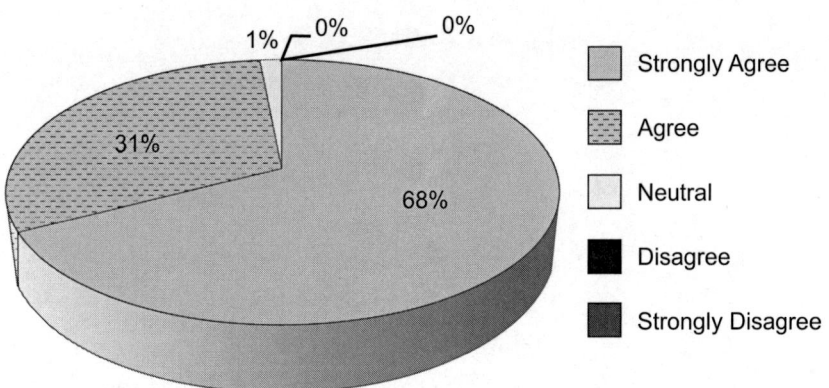

An overwhelming 99 per cent of respondents either strongly agreed or agreed with the statement that there was a need for strong, independent regulation of the professions of nursing and midwifery in

Ireland centred on the protection of the public. This must be seen as an encouraging response and confirmation that, within this target group, the key message of the Act has been understood. If, for example, there had been a desire to retain an element of self-regulation, this would have undoubtedly manifested itself in a higher number of neutral responses (in fact only 1 per cent were neutral) and perhaps also some who either disagreed or strongly disagreed with the statement. There were none.

A question on patient safety elicited a more nuanced response, as can be seen from Figure 3. While 89 per cent of respondents either strongly agreed or agreed with the statement that patient safety was a key driver of professional nursing and midwifery care in Ireland, 8 per cent were neutral and 3 per cent disagreed with the statement. Among the comments made by respondents were the following:

> Patient safety has to be a key priority in the future; patient[s] must be involved in the decision-making process about their health service and their individual care. (NMPDU)

> While patient safety to a degree is a key driver of professional nursing and midwifery care in Ireland, the moratorium on recruitment has compromised patient care and safety. (Director of Nursing)

> Patient safety should be a key driver of professional nursing and midwifery care in Ireland; unfortunately it is economics. (Director of Nursing)

Figure 3: Patient Safety

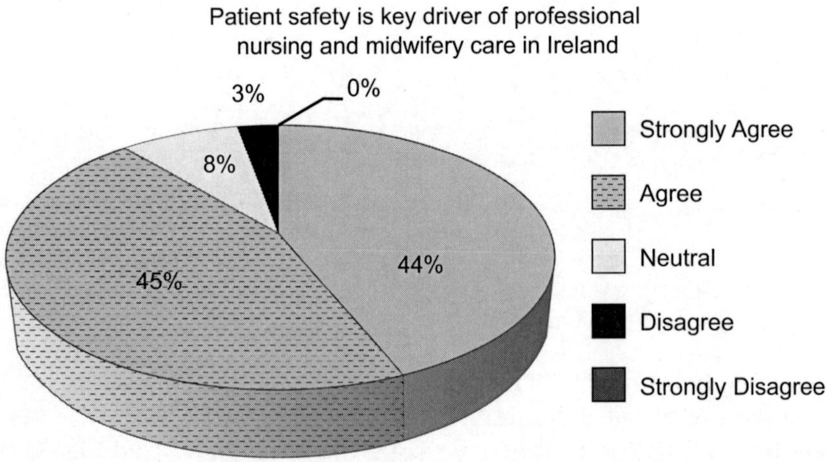

Patient safety is key driver of professional nursing and midwifery care in Ireland

Pressure on the availability of nursing and midwifery resources at the front-line as a result of the Government's moratorium on recruitment and replacement of staff is seen as a threat to patient safety. This is a theme that surfaced a number of times throughout the survey.

Closely linked to patient safety is accountability (Figure 4). In response to the statement that nurses and midwives in Ireland understood and accepted the need for personal legal and professional accountability to their patients, the public, their employer and the regulator, 83 per cent either strongly agreed or agreed, 13 per cent were neutral, 3 per cent disagreed and 1 per cent strongly disagreed. Among the personal comments added by respondents were:

> I don't think all midwives and nurses are fully aware of their personal legal and professional accountability. (CME)

> Professional Accountability – I believe the nursing profession needs to build on this process particularly in relation to developing and maintaining competence; new nurse legislation will support this in context of maintaining a portfolio/evidence of ongoing education/training/professional development. (CNE)

There is some doubt, therefore, about the extent to which accountability is a reality among nurses and midwives and the level of

Figure 4: Professional Accountability

Nurses and midwives in Ireland understand and accept the need for personal legal and professional accountability to their patients, the public, their employer and the regulator

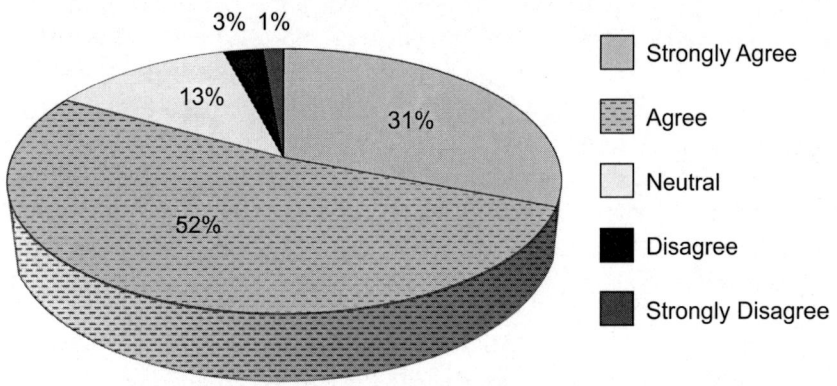

awareness of the implications of the Nurses and Midwives Act 2011 in the area of maintaining and providing evidence of professional competence as an important part of professional accountability.

When asked for their views on the statement that nurses and midwives were aware of and supported the development of guidelines, policies and protocols aimed at ensuring the highest standards in the delivery of care (Figure 5), 89 per cent either strongly agreed or agreed with the statement and 11 per cent were neutral.

Figure 5: Guidelines, Policies and Protocols

Nurses and midwives in Ireland are aware of and support the development of guidelines, policies and protocols aimed at ensuring the highest standards in the delivery of care

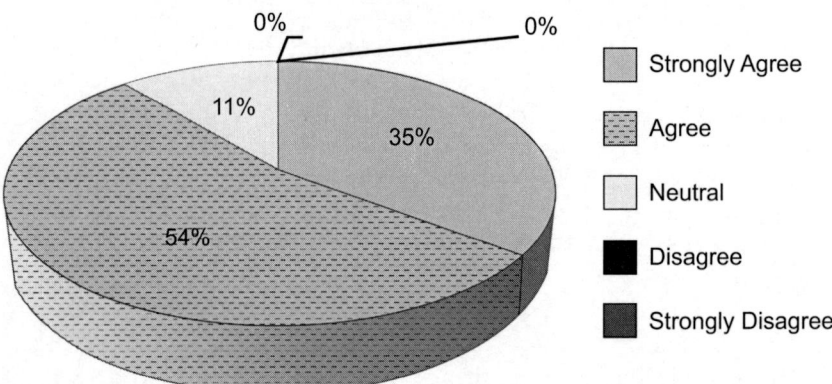

When asked for their views on the statement that nurses and midwives in Ireland understood and accepted the importance of ongoing clinical audits aimed at identifying progress in the achievement of identified outcomes and KPIs (Figure 6), only 15 per cent strongly agreed with the statement, 55 per cent agreed, 20 per cent were neutral, 8 per cent disagreed and 1 per cent strongly disagreed. This reaction is an interesting contrast with the previous question (Figure 5), where there was evidence of a high level of awareness of the need for guidelines, policies and protocols. In this question (Figure 6), there would appear to be less certainty about the need to translate this into a system that verifies compliance and achievement of standards and KPIs. Among the comments were the following:

> The importance of clinical audit is not embraced by all nurses and midwifes. The level of postgraduate education that a

nurse/midwife has undertaken goes a long way in driving audit and research. (Director of Nursing)

Practice development including clinical audit initiatives should be strategically driven and evaluated. (CNE/CME)

It is evident, therefore, that, in practice, there is still ground to be made up in the use of clinical audits in nursing and midwifery.

Figure 6: Clinical Audits

Nurses and midwives in Ireland understand and accept
the importance of ongoing clinical audits aimed at identifying progress
in the achievement of identified outcomes and key performance indicators

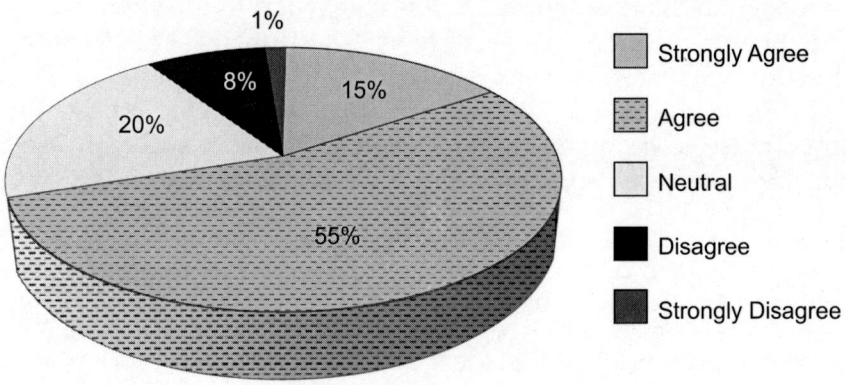

Respondents were also invited to give their opinion on two statements related to the provision of leadership by nurses and midwives in the planning, development and delivery of health services and nursing-/midwifery-led services. The responses are shown in Figures 7 and 8.

Figure 7 shows that almost all (96 per cent) either strongly agreed or agreed with the statement that nurses and midwives in Ireland accept the need to provide leadership in the planning and delivery of healthcare services. Among the comments, two related to the question of the involvement of nurses and midwives at executive level. The development of the executive nurse, as discussed earlier in this book,[442] was reflected in the comments:

Nurses need to become more involved in strategic planning and business planning at an executive level. (Director of Nursing)

My response to the above questionnaire reflects my perception of the reality of nursing in Ireland. There should be opportunities for nurses to become leaders of healthcare; however, I do not see evidence of this on the ground. Healthcare remains dominated by a medical model and nurse managers are not involved in strategic areas of policy and organizational management. Unfortunately, nurses do not appear to be able to articulate their expertise and value to the patient, the multidisciplinary team and the organization. This both frustrates and upsets me as a nurse manager. (Director of Nursing)

The last comment indicates that, on the one hand, there is an onus on nurses and midwives themselves to demonstrate that they are capable of making an impact at this level and on the other there is frustration at the continued dominance of the medical model at the executive and strategic level.

Respondents to this question (Figure 7) also emphasised the importance of the national clinical programmes[443] and expressed the desire for more nursing and midwifery involvement:

With the advent of the National Clinical Programmes this will be a good development for the profession of nursing and midwifery. (Director of Midwifery)

Nurses and midwifery leaders could be more involved in the National Clinical Programmes. I feel a Director of Midwifery should be on the Obstetrics and Gynaecology Care Programme

Figure 7: Leadership in Planning and Delivery

Nurses and midwives in Ireland accept the need to provide leadership in the planning and delivery of healthcare services

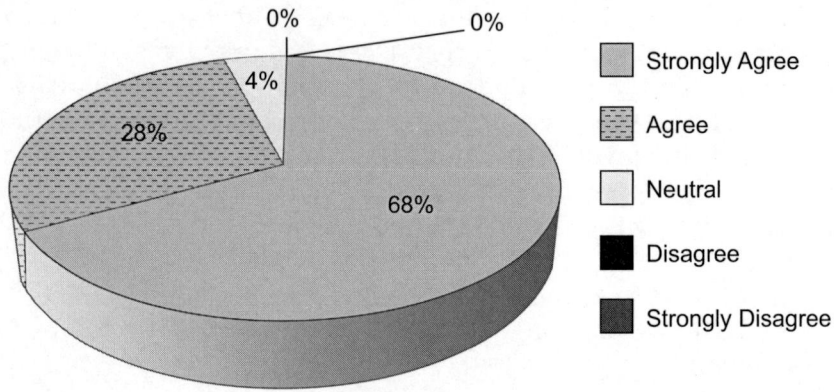

and Neonatal Care Programme and on each implementation group. (CME)

There is an absence of inspirational leaders within Irish nursing. (Director of Nursing)

When asked for their views about whether nurses and midwives in Ireland were increasingly involved in the planning, development and delivery of nursing-/midwifery-led services (Figure 8), 67 per cent either strongly agreed or agreed with the statement, 10 per cent were neutral, 20 per cent disagreed and 3 per cent strongly disagreed. One comment was that:

Nurses and Midwives must be more aware of professionalism in their role. They have a great opportunity to be leaders in the area of nurse-led services and new innovations in healthcare. (NMPDU)

In Figure 9, 82 per cent of respondents either strongly agreed or agreed with the statement that nurses and midwives in Ireland increasingly work as part of an interdisciplinary team in the planning and delivery of care, 7 per cent were neutral, 8 per cent disagreed and 3 per cent strongly disagreed.

Involvement in interdisciplinary teams in the planning and delivery of care is closely related to the theme of integration of health services. There has been a strong movement towards the

Figure 8: Involvement in Nursing- and Midwifery-Led Services

Nurses and midwives in Ireland are increasingly involved in the planning, development and delivery of nursing- and midwifery-led services

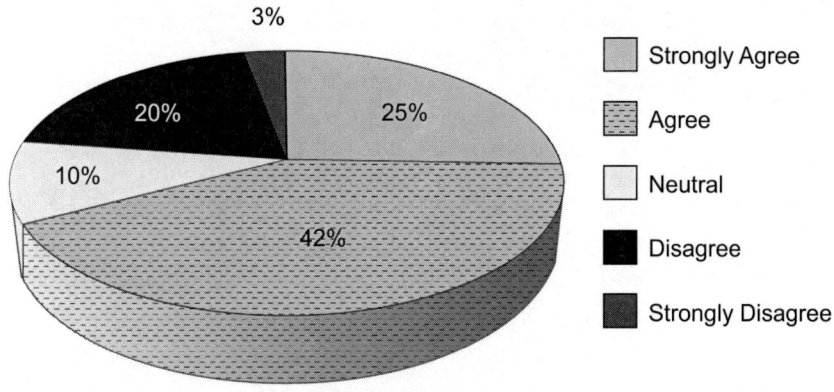

Figure 9: Interdisciplinary Team Planning and Delivery

Nurses and midwives in Ireland increasingly work as part of
an interdisciplinary team in the planning and delivery of care

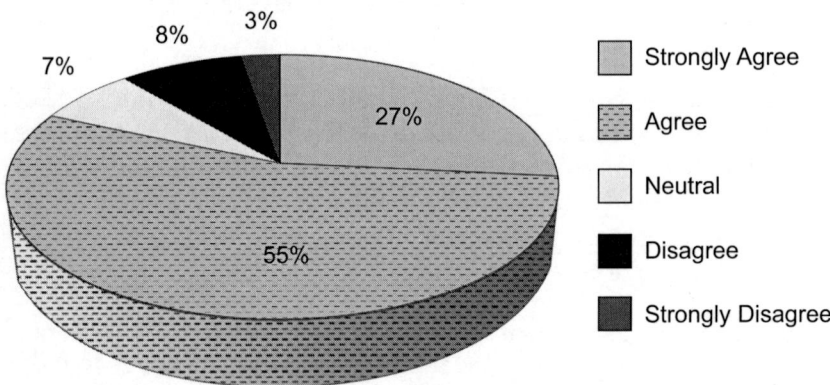

breaking-down of barriers between acute and community-based care in Ireland in recent years. Figure 10 contains the views of the respondents on the statement that healthcare in Ireland was rapidly moving towards a model of integrated care. Only 10 per cent of respondents strongly agreed with this statement and 42 per cent agreed. A large proportion (48 per cent) were either neutral (30 per cent), disagreed (17 per cent) or strongly disagreed (1 per cent). Some expressed their frustration at the slow pace of integration:

Figure 10: Integrated Care

Healthcare delivery in Ireland is rapidly moving
towards a model of integrated care

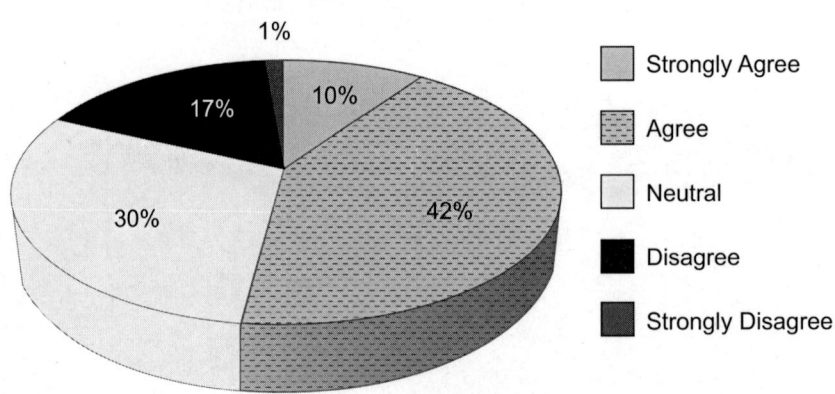

Integration is slow and tedious. (Director of Nursing)

Though work is under way (in the context of the transformational programme and clinical care programmes) to build resources and infrastructure, I believe there needs to be greater urgency and emphasis on developing integrated services in the community, as this is where nurses (particularly CNS, ANP roles) can have the greatest impact on patient/client outcomes. There is still too much emphasis on acute care and the medical model of care – needs to be balanced. (CNE)

While healthcare delivery in Ireland should be rapidly moving towards a model of integrated care, there is significant disempowerment of key personnel to drive or enable integration. (Director of Nursing)

A true integrated model of care will become more evident if the structures and/or processes to facilitate this are developed and implemented. The fact that we have a two-tier health system (public and private) both in primary care and in the secondary care sector does not support integration either. (NMPDU)

There was further evidence of frustration at the slow pace of integration in Figure 11, where respondents were asked for their views on the statement that there was strong evidence of increased links between acute and community care settings in nursing and midwifery in Ireland. Only 3 per cent of respondents strongly agreed with this statement and 34 per cent agreed. The majority (63 per cent) were either neutral (30 per cent), disagreed (30 per cent) or strongly disagreed (3 per cent). Here are some comments:

A lot of work is required to establish links between the acute hospitals and community. (Director of Nursing)

Whilst there is evidence for increased links between nurses and midwives who work in the community and their colleagues in the hospitals, it appears that it is often ad hoc rather than structured. Given that there are separate budgets and staff reporting relationships – these do not support real improved links. We don't yet have PHNs based in EDs whose roles are to assess and facilitate early discharge/prevent admission. (NMPDU)

Figure 11: Links Between Acute and Community Care

There is strong evidence of increased links between acute and
community care settings in nursing and midwifery in Ireland

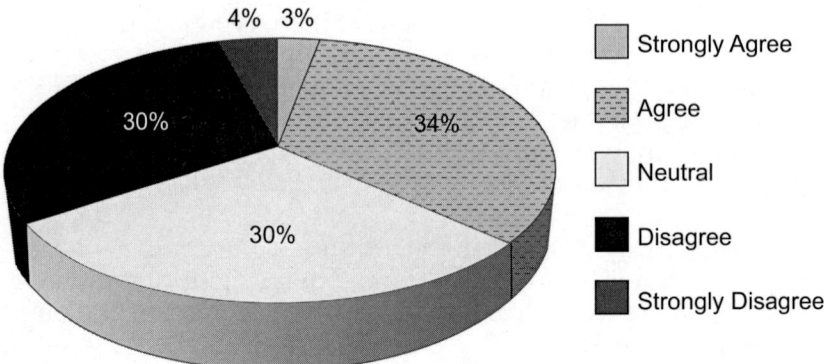

Change in the expectations that more services can be delivered
in the Community is leading to greater integration of Nursing
& Midwifery and the development of links across the care
settings. (Director of Nursing)

When asked for their views on the statement that more and more
nursing and midwifery care in Ireland was being delivered in
community settings (Figure 12), 6 per cent strongly agreed and 39
per cent agreed. A large number (54 per cent) were either neutral
(31 per cent), disagreed (15 per cent) or strongly disagreed (8 per cent).

Figure 12: Nursing and Midwifery Care in the Community

More and more nursing and midwifery care in Ireland
is being delivered in community settings

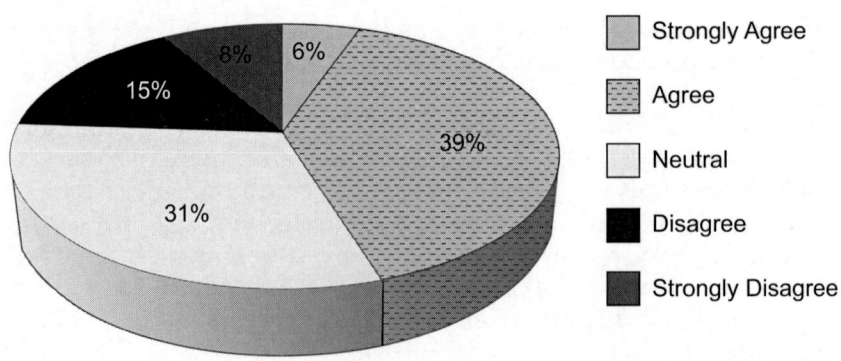

Comments showed frustration at the slowness of developments in this area and, on the other hand, a sense of disempowerment at not being able to make decisions or be involved in key decision-making in this area:

> Care in the community needs to increase its pace in line with expanded roles and acuity. (Director of Nursing)

> Nurses and Midwifes in senior management positions are curtailed from the decision-making process most especially in respect of nurse management in the community. They are responsible and accountable largely for implementing policies which have been developed without their expertise or without consultation with them. There is a void at senior level in terms of expert knowledge of community nursing and an apparent lack of understanding of the need to engage with the expertise available. At a time when more is needed and demanded from the community services, this situation very badly needs to be dealt [with]. (Director of Public Health Nursing)

> Re 'more and more nursing care in the community' – unfortunately this largely remains an aspiration with a few exceptions. (NMPDU)

> Nurses in the community setting are not embracing the opportunities. In addition much of nursing development is still centred on a hospital model and not community etc! (Director of Nursing)

> Primary Care to be a reality, not just talked about. (Director of Nursing)

On the key question of expansion of practice and awareness of the availability of guidance,[444] respondents were asked for their views on the statement that there existed a clear strategic framework and clear guidelines for the expansion of the roles of nurses and midwives in Ireland (Figure 13); 62 per cent either strongly agreed or agreed with this statement. A large proportion were either neutral (20 per cent) or disagreed (18 per cent). These results are surprising in that the respondents represent the senior leaders of the profession and one could have expected a stronger endorsement of the guidelines and frameworks that are in place. Perhaps this is indicative of

Figure 13: Guidelines for Expansion of Roles

There exists a clear strategic framework and clear guidelines for the expansion of the roles of nurses and midwives in Ireland

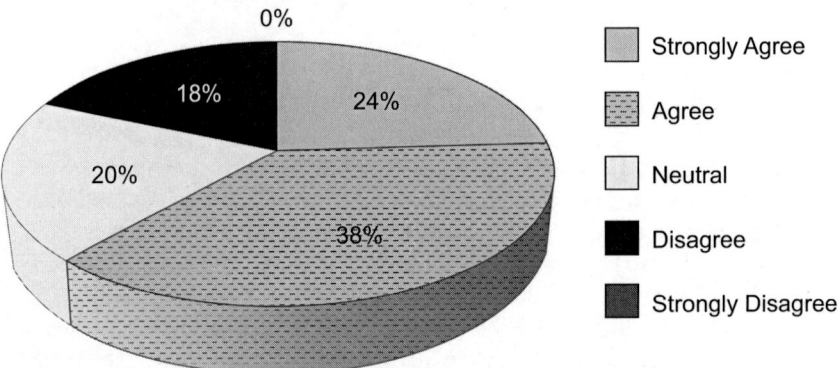

the need for more awareness-raising among this cohort of what is available and the development of a greater understanding of how the guidelines and frameworks should be used. Comments show a positive disposition towards the frameworks and some frustration at resistance to change in some quarters within the professions:

> The Scope of Practice Framework provides an excellent tool for role expansion and development of Clinical Care pathways. (CME)

> Nurses are still reluctant to take on some expanded roles (within scope of nursing practice framework) – unfortunately, even when in the best interest of patients and the service, staff shortages/skill mix issues ha[ve] given justification to this mindset even among nurse managers. (CNE)

Respondents were asked for their views on the statement that the roles of nurses and midwives in Ireland were expanding in line with the needs of patients and of the services (Figure 14). 72 per cent either strongly agreed (18 per cent) or agreed (54 per cent), while 14 per cent were neutral and 14 per cent disagreed.

The survey contained two questions related to education, one on undergraduate education and one on postgraduate education. Respondents were asked for their views on the statement that undergraduate education for nurses and midwives in Ireland prepared them well for the challenges they faced as professionals (Figure 15).

Figure 14: Expansion of Roles in Line with the Needs of Patients and Services

The roles of nurses and midwives in Ireland are expanding in line with the needs of patients and of the services

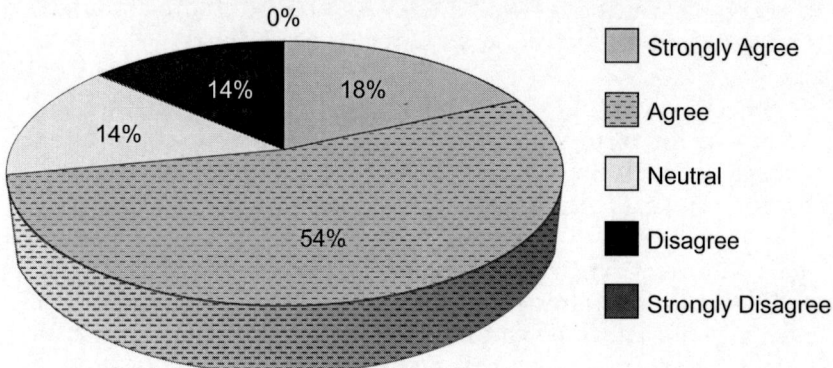

48 per cent either strongly agreed (10 per cent) or agreed (38 per cent). Most (53 per cent) were either neutral (24 per cent), disagreed (23 per cent) or strongly disagreed (6 per cent). Given the large investment that has been made in nursing and midwifery education since the *Report of the Commission on Nursing*[445] and in view of the fact that the Department of Health has launched a review of undergraduate education for nurses and midwives,[446] these findings are interesting. The comments made by respondents help to add some nuance to the responses and highlight some of the issues that need to be addressed as part of a review of undergraduate education. In general, there is evidence that respondents are enthusiastic about and welcome the undergraduate programme and want it to continue. However, they also identify the need for some changes in order to ensure that the appropriate competencies are developed and that students gain access to the kind of education they require to meet the challenges of nursing and midwifery care:

> The undergraduate programme should continue; the review should favour the excellent results it's currently achieving in preparing nurses for the future. (Director of Nursing)

> I enthusiastically welcome the review of undergraduate education. (NMPDU)

> More emphasis needs to be placed on leadership at undergraduate level and an emphasis on clinical nurse leaders as

role models and mentors, for those without leadership experience, at clinical level. (Director of Nursing)

I welcome the direct entry programme. My experience of the direct entry midwives working at (my hospital) are confident and competent practitioners. (Director of Nursing)

The need to expand community experience for students is a key need for future; at present opportunities for community experience is limited but necessary if they are to be prepared for the future. (Third level)

This comment particularly relates to psychiatric nursing and intellectual disability nursing. In my opinion psychiatric nursing preparation requires an increased focus on clinical risk assessment and management of the recovery model. Intellectual disability nursing requires a greater focus on providing a social model of care and the role of the nurse in this clinical context. (NMPDU)

I also have some generic concerns about the structure of clinical placements and roles adopted prior to internship (the role adopted by students when 'supernumerary'). The former results in students not gaining any exposure to the main aspects of care (medical/surgical nursing) for a long period during the programme – resulting in a potential loss of knowledge and skill – and these have to be re-taught later in the programme.

Figure 15: Undergraduate Education

Undergraduate education for nurses and midwives in Ireland prepares them well for the challenges they face as professionals

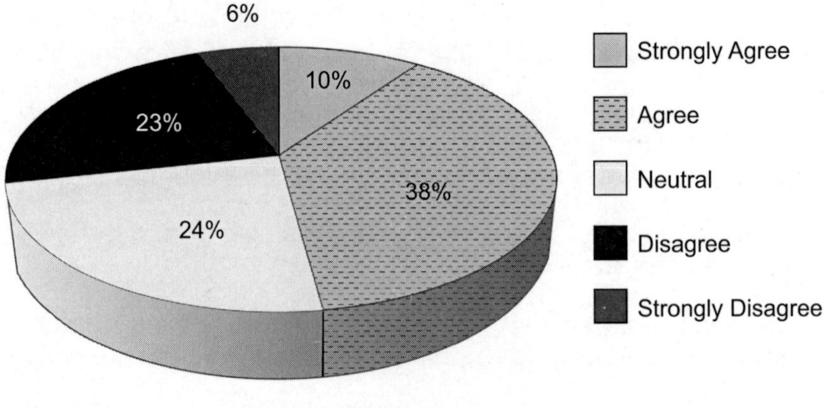

- 6%
- 10%
- 23%
- 24%
- 38%

Strongly Agree
Agree
Neutral
Disagree
Strongly Disagree

The latter can result in the creation of a lack of identification with a specific clinical area and can result in a lack of real engagement with nursing and therefore the embedding of the application of the theory gained to clinical practice. (NMPDU)

Furthermore I don't think there is enough theory provided or processes in place to ensure that students are competent in undertaking a full nursing assessment, care planning and other aspects of the 'nursing process' (all undergrad programmes). (NMPDU)

There is also not enough emphasis on how to demonstrate 'caring' and 'compassion' in clinical practice – what are the behaviours/approach/speech content that a nurse requires to be seen to demonstrate these qualities. (NMPDU)

There is a need to develop an undergraduate nursing curriculum to reflect the changing role of Nurses and Midwives. (CNE/CME)

On postgraduate education (Figure 16), respondents were asked for their views on the statement that postgraduate and continuous professional development opportunities for nurses and midwives in Ireland prepared them well for the development of their roles in the healthcare services; 80 per cent of respondents either strongly agreed (18 per cent) or agreed (62 per cent), while 8 per cent were

Figure 16: Postgraduate Education

Postgraduate education and continuous professional development opportunities for nurses and midwives in Ireland prepare them well for the development of their roles in the healthcare services

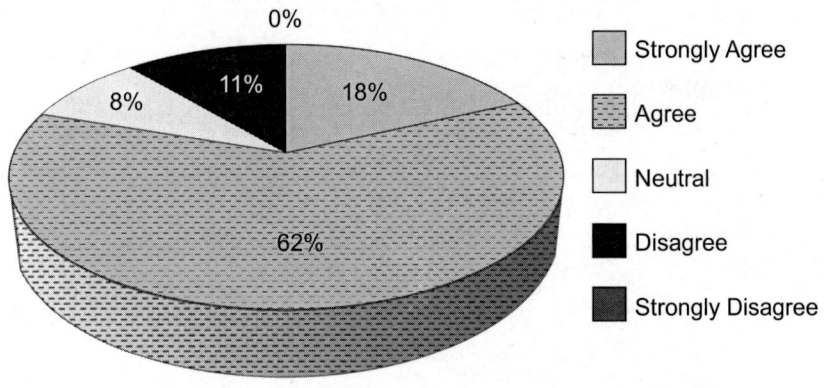

neutral and 11 per cent disagreed. The response to this question is an endorsement of the considerable amount of development that has taken place in this area in recent years. One comment called for the need for further development in line with the needs of the services:

> Postgraduate education and continuing professional development opportunities should be further tailored to meet the need[s] of services. (CNME)

The final survey question (Figure 17) related to career pathways. Respondents were asked for their views on the statement that nurses and midwives in Ireland have a wide and professionally rewarding clinical career pathway; 67 per cent either strongly agreed (18 per cent) or agreed (49 per cent), while 17 per cent were neutral, 13 per cent disagreed and 3 per cent strongly disagreed. At a time when nurses and midwives in Ireland are under extreme pressure because of the cutbacks in the health services, the demands for increased outputs and the amount of change that is taking place within the services, these results are encouraging. Despite the challenges of these very difficult times, over two-thirds of respondents were enthusiastic about the career pathways that have been developed since the publication of the *Report of the Commission on Nursing*[447] and this is thanks to the work of the National Council in this area. This was noted in one comment:

Figure 17: Career Pathways

Nurses and midwives in Ireland have a wide and professionally rewarding clinical career pathway

- Strongly Agree
- Agree
- Neutral
- Disagree
- Strongly Disagree

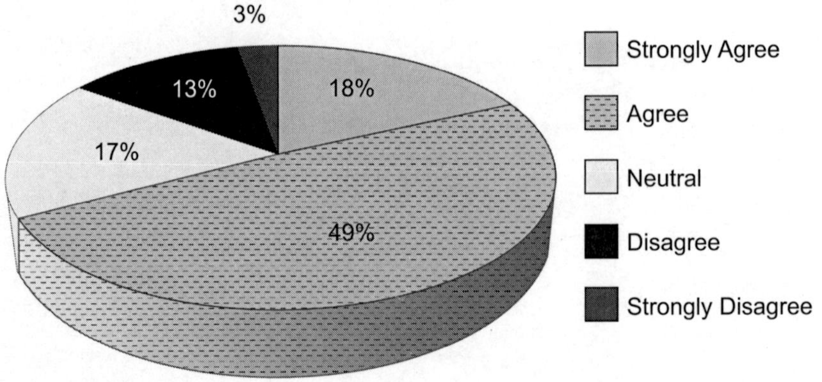

Much of the progress in professional development-practice education, research is due to implementation of recommendations of the Commission on Nursing and vision of the NCNM. (CME)

In these challenging times it is important not to let the standards slip for the professionalism of nurses and midwives, and to ensure roles are protected. (Director of Nursing)

In order to ensure that standards do not slip, especially in times of economic hardship, it is important to be able to fall back on the core values of the professions, the essence of nursing and midwifery. It is these core values that will provide the inspiration for the leaders of the profession and for each and every nurse and midwife to stay true to what it means to be a professional in today's demanding environment.

The Bologna Declaration of 19 June 1999 Joint declaration of the European Ministers of Education

The European process, thanks to the extraordinary achievements of the last few years, has become an increasingly concrete and relevant reality for the Union and its citizens. Enlargement prospects together with deepening relations with other European countries, provide even wider dimensions to that reality. Meanwhile, we are witnessing a growing awareness in large parts of the political and academic world and in public opinion of the need to establish a more complete and far-reaching Europe, in particular building upon and strengthening its intellectual, cultural, social and scientific and technological dimensions.

A Europe of Knowledge is now widely recognised as an irreplaceable factor for social and human growth and as an indispensable component to consolidate and enrich the European citizenship, capable of giving its citizens the necessary competences to face the challenges of the new millennium, together with an awareness of shared values and belonging to a common social and cultural space.

The importance of education and educational cooperation in the development and strengthening of stable, peaceful and democratic societies is universally acknowledged as paramount, the more so in view of the situation in South East Europe.

The Sorbonne declaration of 25th of May 1998, which was underpinned by these considerations, stressed the Universities' central role in developing European cultural dimensions. It emphasised the creation of the European area of higher education as a key way to promote citizens' mobility and employability and the Continent's overall development.

Several European countries have accepted the invitation to commit themselves to achieving the objectives set out in the declaration, by signing it or expressing their agreement in principle. The direction taken by several higher education reforms launched in the meantime in Europe has proved many Governments' determination to act.

European higher education institutions, for their part, have accepted the challenge and taken up a main role in constructing the European area of higher education, also in the wake of the fundamental principles laid down in the Bologna Magna Charta Universitatum of 1988. This is of the highest importance, given that Universities' independence and autonomy ensure that higher education and research systems continuously adapt to changing needs, society's demands and advances in scientific knowledge.

The course has been set in the right direction and with meaningful purpose. The achievement of greater compatibility and comparability of the systems of higher education nevertheless requires continual momentum in order to be fully accomplished. We need to support it through promoting concrete measures to achieve tangible forward steps. The 18th June meeting saw participation by authoritative experts and scholars from all our countries and provides us with very useful suggestions on the initiatives to be taken.

We must in particular look at the objective of increasing the international competitiveness of the European system of higher education. The vitality and efficiency of any civilisation can be measured by the appeal that its culture has for other countries. We need to ensure that the European higher education system acquires a world-wide degree of attraction equal to our extraordinary cultural and scientific traditions.

While affirming our support to the general principles laid down in the Sorbonne declaration, we engage in coordinating our policies to reach in the short term, and in any case within the first decade of the third millennium, the following objectives, which we consider to be of primary relevance in order to establish the European area of higher education and to promote the European system of higher education world-wide:

Adoption of a system of **easily readable and comparable degrees**, also through the implementation of the diploma supplement, in order to promote European citizens' employability and the international competitiveness of the European higher education system.

Adoption of a system essentially based on **two main cycles**, undergraduate and graduate. Access to the second cycle shall require successful completion of first cycle studies, lasting a minimum of three years. The degree awarded after the first cycle shall also be relevant to the European labour market as an appropriate level of qualification. The second cycle should lead to the master and/or doctorate degree as in many European countries.

Establishment of a **system of credits** – such as in the ECTS system – as a proper means of promoting the most widespread student mobility. Credits could also be acquired in non-higher education contexts, including lifelong learning, provided they are recognised by receiving Universities concerned.

Promotion of **mobility** by overcoming obstacles to the effective exercise of free movement with particular attention to:

- for students, access to study and training opportunities and to related services
- for teachers, researchers and administrative staff, recognition and valorisation of periods spent in a European context researching, teaching and training, without prejudicing their statutory rights.

Promotion of **European cooperation in quality assurance** with a view to developing comparable criteria and methodologies.

Promotion of the **necessary European dimensions in higher education**, particularly with regards to curricular development, inter-institutional cooperation, mobility schemes and integrated programmes of study, training and research.

We hereby undertake to attain these objectives – within the framework of our institutional competences and taking full respect of the diversity of cultures, languages, national education systems and of University autonomy – to consolidate the European area of higher education. To that end, we will pursue the ways of intergovernmental cooperation, together with those of non-governmental European organisations with competence on higher education. We expect Universities again to respond promptly and positively and to contribute actively to the success of our endeavour.

Convinced that the establishment of the European area of higher education requires constant support, supervision and adaptation to the continuously evolving needs, we decide to meet again within two years in order to assess the progress achieved and the new steps to be taken.

Survey of Nursing and Midwifery, December 2011

Yvonne O'Shea
Chief Executive Officer
National Council for the Professional Development of
Nursing and Midwifery
Email: yoshea@ncnm.ie

This survey is being carried out as part of a wider research exercise. The results of the survey will be aggregated and the identity of individual respondents will not be released. You are asked to place an 'x' in the box that most accurately reflects your view of the statement contained in the left-hand column. The box at the end of the survey questionnaire is for you to add any additional comments you may wish to make.

Please email your response as an attachment by replying to the email in which this document arrived. Please return completed forms on or before 12th December 2011.

Your cooperation and participation is greatly appreciated. The results of the survey and of the wider research will be made available during the first half of 2012.

	Strongly Agree	Agree	Neutral	Disagree	Strongly Disagree
Nurses and midwives in Ireland accept the need to provide leadership in the planning and delivery of healthcare services.					

	Strongly Agree	Agree	Neutral	Disagree	Strongly Disagree
Nurses and midwives in Ireland are increasingly involved in the planning, development and delivery of nursing- and midwifery-led services.					
There exists a clear strategic framework and clear guidelines for the expansion of the roles of nurses and midwives in Ireland.					
The roles of nurses and midwives in Ireland are expanding in line with the needs of patients and of the services.					
Nurses and midwives in Ireland increasingly work as part of an interdisciplinary team in the planning and delivery of care.					
Healthcare delivery in Ireland is rapidly moving towards a model of integrated care.					
There is strong evidence of increased links between acute and community care settings in nursing and midwifery in Ireland.					
More and more nursing and midwifery care in Ireland is being delivered in community settings.					
Undergraduate education for nurses and midwives in Ireland prepares them well for the challenges they face as professionals.					
Postgraduate education and continuous professional development opportunities for nurses and midwives in Ireland prepare them well for the development of their roles in the healthcare services.					
Nurses and midwives in Ireland have a wide and professionally rewarding clinical career pathway.					
Patient safety is a key driver of professional nursing and midwifery care in Ireland.					

	Strongly Agree	Agree	Neutral	Disagree	Strongly Disagree
There is a need for strong, independent regulation of the professions of nursing and midwifery in Ireland, centred on the protection of the public.					
Nurses and midwives in Ireland understand and accept the need for personal legal and professional accountability to their patients, the public, their employer and the regulator.					
Nurses and midwives in Ireland are aware of and support the development of guidelines, policies and protocols aimed at ensuring the highest standards in the delivery of care.					
Nurses and midwives in Ireland understand and accept the importance of ongoing clinical audits aimed at identifying progress in the achievement of identified outcomes and key performance indicators.					

Additional comments:	
Name (*optional*)	
Organisation	
Branch of the Register	
Job Title	

Thank you for your help.

ENDNOTES

Introduction

1   O'Shea (2008a).
2   O'Shea (2009).
3   Government of Ireland (1998).
4   Department of An Taoiseach (2011).
5   Government of Ireland (2011a).
6   Department of Health (2012a).
7   Department of An Taoiseach (2011).

Chapter 1

8   O'Shea (2008a), Chapter 1.
9   Nightingale (1860).
10   Henderson (1961).
11   World Health Organisation (1996).
12   Kitson (1999).
13   e.g. Benner (1984), Titchen (1998).
14   Rogers (1976).
15   Kitson (1999).
16   Benner (1984), Benner et al. (1999).
17   Kitson (1999).
18   Kitson (1999).
19   Neuman (1995).
20   George (1996).
21   Benner (1984).
22   Orem (1985).
23   Roper, Logan and Tierney (2000).
24   Henderson (1966).
25   Laing (1971).
26   National Council (2008a, 2008b, 2008c).

Chapter 2

27   Department of Health (2011a). Unless otherwise stated, data provided in this section of this chapter is taken from the Department of Health's publication

Health in Ireland: Key Trends 2011 (www.dohc.ie/publications/key_trends_
2011).

28   Central Statistics Office (2012a).
29   Department of Health (2012b).
30   Central Statistics Office (2012a).
31   Total fertility rate (TFR) is a measure of the average number of children a
      woman could expect to have if the fertility rates for a given year pertained
      throughout her fertile years (Department of Health, 2011a).
32   World Health Organisation (2010).
33   Age-standardised mortality rates, which are based on a standard European
      population, allow for comparison between years or regions by taking account
      of different proportions of people in the various age categories (Department of
      Health, 2011a).
34   *Irish Times* (2012a).
35   National Suicide Research Foundation (2012a, 2012b).
36   http://www.dohc.ie/statistics/key_trends/health_of_the_population/
      figure_2-7.html.
37   Foley (2012).
38   *Irish Times* (2012b).
39   Health Research Board (2012).
40   Giovino et al. (2012).
41   Economic and Social Research Institute/Trinity College Dublin (2012), http://
      www.growingup.ie/.
42   Royal College of Physicians of Ireland National Immunisation Advisory
      Committee (2008).
43   Government of Ireland (1970).
44   Department of Health (1994).
45   Department of Health (1986).
46   World Health Organisation (1981).
47   Commission on Health Funding (1989).
48   Kennedy (1991).
49   Department of Health (1990a).
50   Department of Health and Children (2001a).
51   Department of Health and Children (2003a).
52   Commission on Financial Management and Control Systems in the Health
      Service (2003).
53   Department of Health and Children (2001b).
54   Department of Health and Children (2002).
55   Department of Health and Children (2004a).
56   ·Prospectus Strategy Consultants (2003).
57   Department of Health and Children (2003b).
58   Health Service Executive (2008a).
59   Government of Ireland (2004a).
60   Government of Ireland (2004a).
61   Health Service Executive (2008a).
62   Office for Health Management (2001a, 2001b, 2002a, 2002b, 2003).
63   Health Service Executive (2005a).
64   O'Shea (2009).

65 Health Service Executive (2006).
66 Health Service Executive (2008a).
67 O'Shea (2009).
68 Health Service Executive (2008a).
69 Health Service Executive (2008b).
70 Health Service Executive (2008c).
71 Health Service Executive (2008d).
72 Department of Health and Children (2008a).
73 Harding Clarke (2006).
74 Department of Health and Children (2008a).
75 www.patientsafetyfirst.gov.ie.
76 www.patientsafetyfirst.gov.ie.
77 Health Information and Quality Authority (2008).
78 Health Information and Quality Authority (2010a).
79 Government of Ireland (2007b).
80 Health Information and Quality Authority (2012a).
81 Health Information and Quality Authority (2012b).
82 Health Information and Quality Authority (2012c).
83 Department of Health (2012c).
84 Health Service Executive (2008a).
85 Health Service Executive (2009a).
86 Health Service Executive (2009b).
87 Health Service Executive (2012a).
88 Health Service Executive (2011a).
89 Health Service Executive (2012b).
90 Health Service Executive (2012a).
91 Department of An Taoiseach (2011), http://www.taoiseach.gov.ie/eng/
    Publications/Publications_Archive/Publications_2011/Programme_for_
    Government_2011.pdf.
92 Government of Ireland (2011b).
93 Department of Health (2012d).
94 Department of Health (2011b).
95 National Treatment Purchase Fund (2010).
96 Department of Health (2011c).
97 Department of Health (2012e).
98 Department of Health (2012e).
99 Department of Health and Children (2006a).
100 Health Service Executive (2005b).
101 Government of Ireland (2001).
102 Government of Ireland (2012a).
103 United Nations (2006).
104 Department of Health (2012f).
105 Government of Ireland (2012a).
106 Department of Health (2011d).
107 Department of Health (2011d).
108 Department of Health (2012g).
109 Department of Health (2012h).
110 Government of Ireland (2004a).

[111] Department of Health (2012i).
[112] Health Service Executive (2012a).
[113] Government of Ireland (2012b).
[114] Department of Health (2012j).
[115] Department of Health (2012k).
[116] Department of Health (2012j).
[117] Department of Health (2012j).
[118] Department of Health (2012l).
[119] Department of Health (2012m).

Chapter 3

[120] Government of Ireland (1919).
[121] Government of Ireland (1950), Government of Ireland (1961a), Government of Ireland (1985).
[122] Government of Ireland (1998).
[123] Government of Ireland (1998).
[124] Government of Ireland (2011a).
[125] Government of Ireland (2011c).
[126] Government of Ireland (2007a).
[127] Government of Ireland (2005a).
[128] Department of Health and Children (2010a).
[129] Department of Health and Children (2001a).
[130] Department of Health and Children (2008a).
[131] Government of Ireland (1985).
[132] Department of Health and Children (2010a).
[133] Department of Health and Children (2010a).
[134] Government of Ireland (1998).
[135] Nurses and Midwives Act 2011, part 10, article 84, paras. 1 to 6, and article 85, paras. 1 to 8.
[136] Government of Ireland (2008).
[137] European Commission (2005a).
[138] National Council (2008a, 2008b, 2008c).
[139] Brook and Rushforth (2011).
[140] Pulcini et al. (2010).
[141] Donald et al. (2010).
[142] Begley et al. (2012).
[143] Kennedy et al. (2012).
[144] Coster et al. (2006), Sheer and Wong (2008).
[145] An Bord Altranais (2010a).
[146] Nurses and Midwives Act 2011, part 2, s. 14.
[147] Nurses Act 1985, part 2, s. 9.
[148] Government of Ireland (2012c).
[149] Nurses Act 1985, part 8, ss. 62 and 63.
[150] An Bord Altranais (2012a).
[151] Department of Health (2011a).
[152] An Bord Altranais (2012a).

[153] An Bord Altranais (2005a, 2005b).
[154] http://www.nursingboard.ie/competency/comp2/domains.asp?show=1#1.
[155] This definition of a midwife was adopted by the ICM and FIGO in 1972 and 1973 respectively and was later adopted by WHO. The definition was amended by the ICM in 1990 and the amendment ratified by FIGO and the WHO in 1991 and 1992 respectively.
[156] This definition was revised and adopted by the ICM Council on 15 June 2011.
[157] An Bord Altranais (2005b).
[158] Government of Ireland (2011a).
[159] An Bord Altranais (2005a).
[160] Department of Health (1984a).
[161] Sheridan (2000).
[162] Department of Health and Children (2006a).
[163] An Bord Altranais (2005a).
[164] Commission of Enquiry on Mental Handicap (1965).
[165] Chavasse (2000).
[166] An Bord Altranais (2004).
[167] An Bord Altranais (2005a).
[168] Kelleher and Musgrave (2000).
[169] An Bord Altranais (2004).
[170] National Council (2003a).
[171] An Bord Altranais (2012a).
[172] Hanafin et al. (2002).
[173] National Council (2003a).
[174] Hanafin et al. (2002).
[175] National Council (2003a).
[176] An Bord Altranais (2004).
[177] An Bord Altranais (2005c).

Chapter 4

[178] Government of Ireland (1998).
[179] Government of Ireland (1998).
[180] An Bord Altranais (1994).
[181] Tyrrell (1998).
[182] Hart (1985).
[183] Government of Ireland (2000).
[184] An Bord Altranais (2005a, 2005b, 2012b).
[185] An Bord Altranais (2012b).
[186] An Bord Altranais (2012b).
[187] An Bord Altranais (2012b).
[188] www.nursingcareers.ie.
[189] An Bord Altranais (2007a, 2007b, 2007c, 2010b, 2012c).
[190] An Bord Altranais (2008).
[191] National Council (2008a, 2008b, 2008c).
[192] Nurses and Midwives Act 2011, part 11, ss. 87 to 91.
[193] National Council (2003a).

[194] National Council (2004a), Medel-Anonuevo et al. (2001).
[195] Health Service Executive (2007).
[196] Nurses and Midwives Act 2011, part 11, s. 90.
[197] National Council (2009a).
[198] National Council (2010a).
[199] National Council (2003a).
[200] National Council (2004a).
[201] National Council (2005a).
[202] Bologna Declaration (1999).
[203] An Bord Altranais (2005d).
[204] An Bord Altranais (2012b).
[205] Department of Health (2012a), http://www.dohc.ie/issues/nmr/.
[206] Department of Health (2012n).
[207] Higher Education Authority (2012).
[208] Aiken et al. (2000).
[209] Begley et al. (2010).
[210] Bologna Declaration (1999).
[211] Bologna Declaration (1999).
[212] An Bord Altranais (2009a).
[213] European Commission (2011).
[214] Mernagh (2010).
[215] National Qualification Authority Ireland (2010).
[216] The Socrates programme was an educational initiative of the European Commission; 31 countries took part. The initial Socrates programme ran from 1994 until 31 December 1999, when it was replaced by the Socrates II programme on 24 January 2000, which ran until 2006. This, in turn, was replaced by the Lifelong Learning Programme 2007–2013, http://ec.europa.eu/education/lifelong-learning-programme/doc78_en.htm.
[217] National Qualification Authority Ireland (2010).
[218] Lokhoff et al. (2010).
[219] Mernagh (2010).
[220] Mernagh (2010).
[221] Fleming and Holmes (2005).
[222] World Health Organisation (2001a, 2009).
[223] Heath (2002).
[224] World Health Organisation (2009).
[225] World Health Organisation (2009).

Chapter 5

[226] Labour Court (1997).
[227] Government of Ireland (1998).
[228] Government of Ireland (1985).
[229] St James's Hospital (1996).
[230] Working Party on General Nursing (1980).
[231] National Council (2008a, 2008b, 2008c).
[232] Department of Health and Children (1999a).

233 MacLellan (2007).
234 MacLellan (2007).
235 Government of Ireland (2010).
236 An Bord Altranais (2010a).
237 Government of Ireland (1988, 2003).
238 Benner (1984).
239 Benner (1984).
240 National Council (2008a).
241 National Council (2008b, 2008c).
242 National Council (2008a, 2008b, 2008c).
243 National Council (2005b, 2008d).
244 National Council (2006a).
245 National Council (2007a).
246 National Council (2008e).
247 National Council (2005c).
248 Office for Health Management (2004).
249 Office for Health Management (2004).
250 National Council (2008f).
251 National Council (2006b).
252 Department of Health and Children (2003c).
253 National Council (2005d).
254 National Council (2006b).
255 Department of Health and Children (2003c).
256 Department of Health and Children (2009a).
257 National Council (2005e).
258 Leahy-Warren and Tyrrell (1998).
259 National Council (2004b).
260 National Council (2005f).
261 Begley et al. (2010).
262 Begley et al. (2010), p. 48.
263 Begley et al. (2010, pp. 49–51), Elliott et al. (2012), Begley et al. (2012).
264 Begley et al. (2012).
265 An Bord Altranais (2000a, 2000c).
266 An Bord Altranais (2000c).
267 An Bord Altranais (2000a, 2000b).
268 Department of Health and Children (2011a).
269 National Council (2009b).
270 National Council (2006c).
271 An Bord Altranais (2000a).
272 Higgins et al. (2010).
273 An Bord Altranais (2000d), Department of Health and Children (2008a), National Council (2009c), National Institute for Health and Clinical Excellence (2007).
274 Health Information and Quality Authority (2010b), National Council (2010b, 2010c).
275 Department of Health and Children (2011a).
276 Department of Health (1997).
277 North Eastern Health Board (2001).

[278] Government of Ireland (1998).
[279] Community Midwifery Service, National Maternity Hospital (2001).
[280] Department of Health and Children (2011a).

Chapter 6

[281] Department of Health (2011a). Tables 10, 11 and 12 are adapted from the HSE's Health Service Personnel Census at 31 December (except for 2011 – see note (v) below) as quoted in *Health in Ireland: Key Trends 2011* (Department of Health, 2011a).

    i.   Figures refer to whole-time equivalents excluding staff on career break. Data also exclude home helps.

    ii.   Caution should be exercised in making grade category comparisons due to changes in category composition over time.

    iii.   'Management/administration' includes staff who are of direct service to the public and include consultants' secretaries, outpatient departmental personnel, medical records personnel, telephonists and other staff who are engaged in front-line duties.

    iv.   Student nurses are included in the 2007 and 2008 employment figures on the basis of 3.5 students equating to 1 whole-time equivalent. The employment levels adjusted for student nurses on the above basis are 110,664 WTE (Dec 2007) and 111,001 WTE (Dec 2008). Student nurses are included in the 2009–2011 figures on the basis of 2 students equating to 1 whole-time equivalent – the figures above are already adjusted.

    v.   The 2011 data refers to September 2011 employment figures. Caution should be exercised in comparing this data to previous years which refer to December figures.

[282] The table in the document *Key Trends* does not distinguish between nursing and midwifery.
[283] World Health Organisation (2010).
[284] World Health Organisation (2010).
[285] World Health Organisation (2010).
[286] World Health Organisation (2010).
[287] Health Service Executive and Irish Hospice Foundation (2008), www.hse.ie and www.hospice-foundation.ie.
[288] Health Service Executive (2012a).
[289] Department of An Taoiseach (2011).
[290] Health Service Executive (2012a).
[291] Health Service Executive et al. (2010).
[292] Health Service Executive et al. (2012).
[293] Department of Health and Children (2006b).
[294] Department of Health (2012o).
[295] Department of Health (2012o).
[296] Department of Health (2011a).
[297] Byrne et al. (2011).
[298] KPMG (2008).

299 Health Service Executive (2012c).
300 KPMG (2008).
301 KPMG (2008).
302 Health Service Executive (2005c).
303 Begley et al. (2009).
304 Begley et al. (2009).
305 Hatem et al. (2008), Devane et al. (2010), Hollowell et al. (2011).
306 Institute of Obstetricians and Gynaecologists (2006).
307 Department of Health and Children (2011a).
308 Harding Clark (2006).
309 Health Service Executive (2012a).
310 Department of An Taoiseach (2011).
311 Government of Ireland (2001).
312 United Nations (2008).
313 Department of Health (2012f).
314 Government of Ireland (2012a).
315 Department of Health (2012p).
316 Department of Health (1984a).
317 Department of Health and Children (2006a).
318 Department of Health and Children (2006a).
319 Health Service Executive (2012d).
320 Department of Health and Children (2006a).
321 Department of Health (2011e).
322 Mental Health Commission (2012).
323 Department of Health (2012q).
324 Mental Health Commission (2007).
325 Dooley and Fitzgerald (2012).
326 McGorry (2005).
327 Hickey (2004), Kessler et al. (2005), Kim-Cohen et al. (2003).
328 Kelly and Kelly (2011).
329 Kelly and Kelly (2011).
330 Department of Health and Children (2009b).
331 Expert Reference Group on Disability Policy (2011).
332 Department of Health (2012r).
333 Health Service Executive (2011b).
334 Department of Health (1990b).
335 Department of Health (1996).
336 Commission on the Status of People with Disabilities (1996).
337 Department of Health and Children (2009b).
338 Health Service Executive (2011b).
339 Health Service Executive (2011b).
340 Health Service Executive (2011b).
341 Health Service Executive (2011b).
342 Department of Environment, Community and Local Government and Department of Health (2012).
343 National Health Service Quality Improvement Scotland (2006).
344 Atherton (2006), Royal College of Nursing (2006).
345 National Health Service (2010).

Endnotes

346 Van Schrojenstein Lantman-de Valk and Noonan Walsh (2008).
347 Felce et al. (2008).
348 Atherton (2006).
349 McCarron et al. (2011).
350 Department of Health and Children (2000a).
351 Department of Health and Children (2010b).
352 Department of Health and Children (2010b).
353 Department of Children and Youth Affairs (2011).
354 Department of Health and Children (2007a).
355 Department of Children and Youth Affairs (2012).
356 *Irish Times* (2012c).
357 In July 2012 HIQA published a guide to national standards for the protection and welfare of children and the national standards for the protection and welfare of children (Health Information and Quality Authority, 2012d, 2012e).
358 Department of An Taoiseach (2011).
359 National Paediatric Hospital Board (2010).
360 National Paediatric Hospital Board (2012).
361 http://www.dcya.gov.ie/.
362 http://www.who.int/healthinfo/survey/ageingdefnolder/en/index.html.
363 Figures based on data from CSO website, http://www.cso.ie/en/releasesand publications/population/populationandlabourforceprojections2006-2036/.
364 Central Statistics Office (2012c).
365 National Council (2007a).
366 Royal College of Nursing and British Geriatrics Society (2001).
367 National Council (2007a).
368 An Bord Altranais (2009b).
369 Health Information and Quality Authority (2009).
370 Health Service Executive (2012a).
371 Health Service Executive and Royal College of Physicians of Ireland (2012).
372 Cahill et al. (2012a).
373 Department of An Taoiseach (2011).
374 Cahill et al. (2012b).
375 Irish Times (2012d).
376 National Council (2007a).
377 O'Shea et al. (2008).
378 World Health Organisation (2011).
379 World Health Organisation (2004a).
380 World Health Organisation (2004b).
381 Health Service Executive and the Irish Hospice Foundation (2008).
382 Department of Health (2012b).
383 Central Statistics Office (2012a).
384 Central Statistics Office (2010).
385 Barret et al. (2011).
386 O'Shea (2009).
387 O'Shea (2009).

Chapter 7

[388] Government of Ireland (2011a).
[389] Government of Ireland (2007a).
[390] Government of Ireland (2005a).
[391] Department of Health (2012c).
[392] Department of Health (2012h).
[393] Department of Health (2012c).
[394] Department of Health (2012c).
[395] Health Information and Quality Authority (2012b).
[396] www.rcsi.ie/noca.
[397] Department of Health and Children (2008a).
[398] www.patientsafetyfirst.gov.ie/.
[399] www.patientsafetyfirst.gov.ie/.
[400] O'Shea (2009).
[401] Health Service Executive (2012e, 2012f).
[402] Health Information and Quality Authority (2012c).
[403] Health Service Executive (2009c).
[404] Department of Health and Children (2008a).
[405] Health Service Executive (2009f).
[406] Health Service Executive (2009c), p. 10.
[407] Health Service Executive (2012e, 2012f).
[408] Health Information and Quality Authority (2012c).
[409] Health Service Executive (2012e, 2012f).
[410] Health Service Executive (2012e, 2012f).
[411] Health Information and Quality Authority (2012c).
[412] Machell et al. (2009), Department of Health (UK) (2006).
[413] Department of Health (2012h).
[414] Carter and Chochinov (2007), Griffin and Melby (2006).
[415] An Bord Altranais (2007a, 2007b, 2007c, 2008, 2010b, 2012c).
[416] Health Service Executive (2012e, 2012f).
[417] Health Service Executive (2012e, 2012f).
[418] www.hse.ie/go/nurseandmidwifeleadership.
[419] International Council of Nurses (2011).
[420] Health Information and Quality Authority (2012c).
[421] Mudiwa (2011).
[422] Department of Health (UK) (2006).
[423] Royal College of Nursing (2005).
[424] Machell et al. (2009).
[425] Royal College of Nursing (2009).
[426] Machell et al. (2009).
[427] Huston (2008).
[428] Mudiwa (2011).
[429] RN4CAST (2012a, 2012b, 2012c).
[430] Begley et al. (2010).
[431] O'Shea (2009).
[432] Health Service Executive (2008e).
[433] O'Shea (2009).

434 Government of Ireland (1998).
435 O'Shea (2009).
436 O'Shea (2009).
437 Government of Ireland (1998).
438 Flynn (1998).
439 Department of Health and Children (2003e).
440 Office for Health Management (2000).
441 Health Information and Quality Authority (2012c).

Chapter 8

442 Machell et al. (2009).
443 Health Service Executive (2012a).
444 An Bord Altranais (2000a, 2000b, 2000c), Department of Health and Children (2011a).
445 Government of Ireland (1998).
446 Department of Health (2012a).
447 Government of Ireland (1998).

REFERENCES

Aiken, L.H., Cimiotti, J.P., Sloane, D.M., Smith, H.L., Flynn, L. and Neff, D.F. (2011), 'Effects of Nurse Staffing and Nurse Education on Patient Deaths in Hospitals with Different Work Environments', *Medical Care*, 49(12): 1047–1053.

Aiken, L.H., Clarke, S.P., Cheung, R.B., Douglas, M.S. and Jeffrey, H.S. (2003), 'Educational Levels and Surgical Patient Mortality', *Journal of the American Medical Association*, 290(12): 1617–1623.

Aiken, L.H., Havens, D.S. and Sloane, D.M. (2000), 'The Magnet Nursing Services Recognition Programme: A Comparison of Two Groups of Magnet Hospitals', *American Journal of Nursing*, 100(3): 26–36.

American Association of Colleges of Nursing (AACN) (2008), 'The Essentials of Baccalaureate Education for Professional Nursing Practice', Washington DC, <http://www.aacn.nche.edu/education/pdf/BaccEssentials08.pdf.>

An Bord Altranais (1994), *The Future of Nurse Education and Training in Ireland*, Dublin: An Bord Altranais.

An Bord Altranais (2000a), *Scope of Nursing and Midwifery Practice Framework*, Dublin: An Bord Altranais.

An Bord Altranais (2000b), *Review of Scope of Practice for Nursing and Midwifery, Final Report*, Dublin: An Bord Altranais.

An Bord Altranais (2000c), *Code of Professional Conduct for each Nurse and Midwife*, Dublin: An Bord Altranais.

An Bord Altranais (2000d), *Guidance on the Development of Policies, Protocols and Guidelines*, Dublin: An Bord Altranais.

An Bord Altranais (2004), *Nurses Rules 2004*, Dublin: An Bord Altranais.

An Bord Altranais (2005a), *Requirements and Standards for Nurse Registration Education Programmes*, 3rd Edition, Dublin: An Bord Altranais.

An Bord Altranais (2005b), *Requirements and Standards for the Midwife Registration Education Programme*, Dublin: An Bord Altranais.

An Bord Altranais (2005c), 'Title Changes to the Division of the Register', *An Bord Altranais News*, 17(1), Dublin: An Bord Altranais.

An Bord Altranais (2005d), 'Five Points Project', Dublin: An Bord Altranais, <http://www.nursingboard.ie/en/spon-five_points.xspx>.

An Bord Altranais (2007a), *Nurses Rules 2007*, Dublin: An Bord Altranais.

References

An Bord Altranais (2007b), *Requirements and Standards for Education Programmes for Nurses and Midwives with Prescriptive Authority*, Dublin: An Bord Altranais.

An Bord Altranais (2007c), *Decision-Making Framework for Nurses and Midwives with Prescriptive Authority*, Dublin: An Bord Altranais.

An Bord Altranais (2008), *Requirements and Standards for Nurse Education Programmes for Authority to Prescribe Ionising Radiation (X-Ray)*, Dublin: An Bord Altranais.

An Bord Altranais (2009a), *Information for Applicants Who Completed Their Training in a European Union (EU) Member State*, Dublin: An Bord Altranais.

An Bord Altranais (2009b), *Professional Guidance for Nurses Working with Older People*, Dublin: An Bord Altranais.

An Bord Altranais (2010a), *Nurses Rules 2010*, Dublin: An Bord Altranais.

An Bord Altranais (2010b), *Practice Standards and Guidelines for Nurses and Midwives with Prescriptive Authority*, Dublin: An Bord Altranais.

An Bord Altranais (2010c), *Guidance for New Nurses and Midwife Registrants*, Dublin: An Bord Altranais.

An Bord Altranais (2010d), *Practice Standards for Midwives*, Dublin: An Bord Altranais.

An Bord Altranais (2010e), *Requirements and Standards for Post-Registration Nursing and Midwifery Education Programmes – Incorporating of the National Framework of Qualifications*, Dublin: An Bord Altranais.

An Bord Altranais (2012a), 'Statistics', <http://www.nursingboard.ie/en/statistics.aspx>.

An Bord Altranais (2012b), *Nursing/Midwifery: A Career for You – Pre-Registration Honours Degree Programmes*, Dublin: An Bord Altranais.

An Bord Altranais (2012c), *Collaborative Practice Agreement for Nurses and Midwives with Prescriptive Authority*, Dublin: An Bord Altranais.

An Bord Altranais and the National Council (National Council for the Professional Development of Nursing and Midwifery) (2005), *Review of Nurses and Midwives in the Prescribing and Administration of Medicinal Products: Final Report*, Dublin: An Bord Altranais and the National Council.

An Bord Altranais and the National Council (National Council for the Professional Development of Nursing and Midwifery) (2008), *Final Report of the Implementation of the Review of Nurses and Midwives in the Prescribing and Administration of Medicinal Products*, Dublin: An Bord Altranais and the National Council.

Antrobus, A. and Kitson, A. (1999), 'Nursing Leadership: Influencing and Shaping Health Policy and Nursing Practice', *Journal of Advance Nursing*, 29(3): 746–753.

Atherton, H. (2006), 'Care Planning for Good Health in Intellectual Disabilities' in B. Gates (ed.), *Care Planning and Delivery in Intellectual Disability Nursing*, Oxford: Blackwell Publishing.

Axelsson, A., Kullen-Engstrom, A. and Edgren, L. (2000), 'Management vs. Symbolic Leadership and Hospitals in Transition: A Swedish Example', *Journal of Nursing Management*, 8: 167–173.

Balanda, K.P., Barron, S., Fahy, A. and McLoughlin, A. (2010), *Making Chronic Disease Count: Hypertension, Stroke, Coronary Heart Disease, Diabetes – A Systematic Approach to Estimating and Forecasting Population Prevalence on the Island of Ireland*, Dublin: Institute of Public Health in Ireland.

Ball, J. (2010), *Guidance on Safe Nurse Staffing Levels in the UK*, London: Royal College of Nursing.

Barr, H. (2003), 'Interprofessional Education: Today, Yesterday and Tomorrow – A Review', commissioned by the Learning and Teaching Support Network for Health Sciences and Practice (LTSN) for the UK Centre for the Advancement of Interprofessional Education (CAIPE), <http://tinyurl.com/m28vnn>.

Barret, A., Savva, G., Tinonen, V. and Kenny, R.A. (2011), *Fifty Plus in Ireland 2011: First Results from the Irish Longitudinal Study on Ageing (TILDA)*, Dublin: Trinity College Dublin.

Barret, G., Sellman, D. and Thomas, J. (eds.) (2005), *Interprofessional Working in Health and Social Care: Professional Perspectives*, Basingstoke: Palgrave Macmillan.

Barrington, R. (2000), *Health, Medicine and Politics in Ireland, 1900–1970*, Dublin: Institute of Public Administration.

Begley, C.M. (2002), '"Great Fleas Have Little Fleas": Irish Student Midwives' Views of the Hierarchy in Midwifery', *Journal of Advanced Nursing*, 38(3): 310–317.

Begley, C., Devane, D. and Clarke, M. (2009), *An Evaluation of Midwifery-Led Care in the Health Service Executive, North Eastern Area: The Report of the MidU Study*, Dublin: Health Service Executive.

Begley, C., Elliott, N., Lalor, J., Coyne, I., Higgins, A. and Comiskey, C.M. (2012), 'Differences between Clinical Specialist and Advanced Practitioner Clinical Practice, Leadership, and Research Roles, Responsibilities, and Perceived Outcomes (the SCAPE Study)', *Journal of Advanced Nursing*, 00(0): 000–000, doi: 10.1111/j.1365-2648.2012.06124.x.

Begley, C., Murphy, K.A., Elliot, N., Lalor, J., Sheerin, F., Coyne, I., Comiskey, C., Normand, C., Casey, C., Dowling, M., Devane, D., Cooney, A., Farrelly, F., Brennan, M., Meskell, P. and MacNeela, P. (2010), *An Evaluation of the Role of the Clinical Nurse/Midwife Specialist and Advanced Nurse/Midwife Practitioner in Ireland: Final Report*, Dublin: National Council.

Begley, C.M., O'Boyle, C., Carroll, M. and Devane, D. (2007), 'Educating Advanced Midwife Practitioners: A Collaborative Venture', *Journal of Nursing Management*, 15: 574–584.

Benner, P. (1984), *From Novice to Expert: Excellence and Power in Clinical Nursing Practice*, Menlo Park, CA: Addison-Wesley Publishing Company.

Benner, P., Hooper-Kyriakidis, P. and Stannard, D. (1999), *Clinical Wisdom and Interventions in Critical Care: A Thinking-in-Action Approach*, Philadelphia, PA: Saunders.

Benner, P., Sutphen, M., Leonard, V. and Day, L. (2010), *Educating Nurses – A Call for Radical Transformation*, San Francisco, CA: Jossey-Bass.

Beveridge, W. (1942), *Social Insurance and Allied Services*, London: Her Majesty's Stationery Office.

Bologna Declaration (1999) 'Joint Declaration of European Ministers of Education. Convened in Bologna on 19th June 1999', <http://www.bologna-bergen2005.no/Docs/00-Main_doc/990719BOLOGNA_DECLARATION.PDF>.

Bower, F.L. (2000), 'Succession Planning: A Strategy for Taking Charge', *Nursing Leadership Forum*, 4(4): 110–113.

Bowles, A. and Bowles, N.B. (2000), 'A Comparative Study of Transformational Leadership in Nursing Development Units and Conventional Clinical Settings', *Journal of Nursing Management*, 8: 69–76.

Buresh, B. and Gordon, S. (2000), *From Silence to Voice: What Nurses Know and Must Communicate to the Public*, Ithaca and London: ILR Press.

Brennan Report *see* Commission on Financial Management and Control Systems in the Health Service.

Brook, S. and Rushforth, H. (2011), 'Why Is the Regulation of Advanced Practice Essential?' *British Journal of Nursing*, 20(16): 996–1000.

Byrne, C., Kennedy, C., O'Dwyer, V., Kennelly, M. and Turner, M.J. (2011), 'What Models of Maternity Care Do Pregnant Women in Ireland Want?', *Irish Medical Journal*, June, 104(6): 180–182.

Cahill, S., O'Shea, E. and Pierce, M. (2012a), *Creating Excellence in Dementia Care: A Research Review for Ireland's National Dementia Strategy*, DSIDC's Living with Dementia Research Programme, School of Social Work and Social Policy, Dublin: Trinity College Dublin, and Galway: Irish Centre for Social Gerontology, National University of Ireland, Galway.

Cahill, S., O'Shea, E. and Pierce, M. (2012b), *Future Dementia Care in Ireland: Sharing the Evidence to Mobilise Action*, DSIDC's Living with Dementia Research Programme, School of Social Work and Social Policy, Dublin: Trinity College Dublin, and Galway: Irish Centre for Social Gerontology, National University of Ireland, Galway.

Carney, M. (1999), 'Leadership in Nursing: Where Do We Go from Here? The Ward Sisters' Challenge for the Future', *Nursing Review*, 17(1/2): 13–18.

Carney, M. (2004), 'Middle Manager Involvement in Strategy Development in Not-for-Profit Organisations: The Director of Nursing Perspective – How Organisational Structure Impacts on the Role', *Journal of Nursing Management*, 12: 13–21.

Carter, A.J.E. and Chocinov, A.H. (2007), 'A Systematic Review of the Impact of Nurse Practitioners on Cost, Quality of Care, Satisfaction and Wait Times in the Emergency Department', *Canadian Journal of Advanced Nursing*, 9(4): 286–995.

Central Statistics Office (2010), *Quarterly National Household Survey (QNHS) – Carers, Quarter 3 2009*, Dublin: Stationery Office.

Central Statistics Office (2012a), *This Is Ireland: Highlights from Census 2011, Part 2*, Dublin: Stationery Office.

Central Statistics Office (2012b), *This Is Ireland: Highlights from Census 2011, Part 1*, Dublin: Stationery Office.

Central Statistics Office (2012c), *Survey on Income and Living Conditions (SILC) – Thematic Report on the Elderly 2004, 2009 and 2010*, Dublin: Stationery Office.

Chavasse, J. (2000), 'Nursing Education', in J. Robins (ed.), *Nursing and Midwifery in Ireland in the Twentieth Century*, Dublin: An Bord Altranais.

Commission of Enquiry on Mental Handicap (1965), *Report of the Commission of Enquiry on Mental Handicap*, Dublin: Government Publications Office.

Commission on Financial Management and Control Systems in the Health Service (2003), *Report of the Commission on Financial Management and Control Systems in the Health Service* (The Brennan Report), Dublin: Stationery Office.

Commission on Health Funding (1989), *Report of the Commission on Health Funding*, Dublin: Stationery Office.

Commission on the Status of People with Disabilities (1996), *A Strategy for Equality: Report of the Commission on the Status of People with Disabilities*, Dublin: National Disability Authority.

Community Midwifery Service, National Maternity Hospital (2001), *The National Maternity Hospital Domino and Hospital Outreach Home Birth Service: Pilot Project Evaluation*, Dublin: Women's Health Unit, Northern Area Health Board.

Condell, S. (1998), *Changes in the Professional Role of Nurses in Ireland: 1980–1997: A Report Prepared for the Commission on Nursing*, Dublin: Stationery Office.

Coster, S., Redfern, S., Wilson-Barnett, J., Evans, A., Peccei, R. and Guest, D. (2006), 'Impact of the Role of Nurse Midwife and Health Visitor Consultant', *Journal of Advanced Nursing*, 55(3): 352–363.

Council of Europe (2003), *Access to Social Rights for People with Disabilities in Europe*, Strasbourg: Council of Europe Publishing.

Council of Europe (2006), *Disability Action Plan 2006–2015*, Strasbourg: Council of Europe.

Council of European Communities (1980), *Council Directive (80/155/EEC) Concerning the Coordination of Provisions Laid down by Law, Regulation or Administrative Action Relating to the Taking up or Pursuit of the Activities of Midwives*, Brussels: Council of European Communities.

Dawould, D. and Maben, J. (2008), *Nurses in Society: Starting the Debate – Writtten Evidence*, National Nursing Research Unit, London: King's College London.

Department of An Taoiseach (2011), 'Programme for Government', <http://www.taoiseach.gov.ie/eng/Publications/Publications_ Archive/Publications_2011/Programme_for_Government_2011.pdf>.

Department of Children and Youth Affairs (2011), *The National Strategy for Research and Data on Children's Lives 2011–2016*, Dublin: Government Publications.

Department of Children and Youth Affairs (2012), *Report of the Independent Child Death Review Group*, Dublin: Government Publications.

Department of Environment, Community and Local Government and the Department of Health (2012), *National Housing Strategy for People with a Disability 2011–2016 – National Implementation Framework*, Dublin: Department of Environment, Community and Local Government and the Department of Health.

Department of Health (1947), 'Outline of Proposals for the Improvement of the Health Services' (White Paper), Dublin: Department of Health.

Department of Health (1971), *SI No 187/1971 – St James's Hospital Board (Establishment) Order, 1971*, Dublin: Stationery Office.

Department of Health (1984a), *The Psychiatric Services: Planning for the Future*, Dublin: Stationery Office.

Department of Health (1984b), *SI No 211/1984 – St James's Hospital Board (Establishment) Order, 1971 (Amendment) Order, 1984*, Dublin: Stationery Office.

Department of Health (1986), *Health: The Wider Dimensions – A Consultative Statement on Policy*, Dublin: Department of Health and Children.

Department of Health (1988), *The Years Ahead: A Policy for the Elderly*, Dublin: Stationery Office.

Department of Health (1990a), *Community Medicine and Public Health: The Future Report of a Working Party Appointed by the Minister for Health* (The Hickey Report), Dublin: Stationery Office.

Department of Health (1990b), *Needs and Abilities: A Policy for the Intellectually Disabled*, Report of the Review Group on Mental Handicap Services, Dublin: Stationery Office.

Department of Health (1994), *Shaping a Healthier Future: A Strategy for Effective Healthcare in the 1990s*, Dublin: Department of Health and Children.

Department of Health (1996), *Towards an Independent Future*, the Review Group on Health and Personal Social Services for People with Physical and Sensory Disabilities, Dublin: Stationery Office.

Department of Health (1997), *A Plan for Women's Health 1997 to 1999*, Dublin: Department of Health.

Department of Health (2011a), *Health in Ireland: Key Trends 2011*, Dublin: Department of Health.

Department of Health (2011b), 'Top International Expert Joins the SDU', press release, 1 June 2011, <http://www.dohc.ie/press/releases/2011/20110601.html>.

Department of Health (2011c), 'Minister Announces Changes in Role of the NTPF to Support the Special Delivery Unit', press release, 28 July 2011, <http://www.dohc.ie/press/releases/2011/20110728.html>.

Department of Health (2011d), 'Cabinet Approves Drafting of Legislation for New HSE Governance', press release, 20 December 2011, <http://www.dohc.ie/press/releases/2011/20111220.html>.

Department of Health (2011e), 'Update on Vision for Change and Mental Health Developments', <http://www.dohc.ie/publications/visionfor change5th/hselocal/hseofficeassistantnatdirectormentalhealth>.

Department of Health (2012a), 'Review of Undergraduate Nursing and Midwifery Degree Programmes', Briefing Paper, 23 February 2012, Dublin: Department of Health.

Department of Health (2012b), *The National Carers' Strategy – Recognised, Supported, Empowered*, Dublin: Department of Health.

Department of Health (2012c), 'Statement from the Minister for Health Following the HIQA Report into Tallaght Hospital', press release, 17 May 2012, <http://www.dohc.ie/press/releases/2012/20120517.html>.

Department of Health (2012d), 'Minister for Health Announces the Establishment of an Implementation Group on Universal Health Insurance', press release, 24 February 2012, <http://www.dohc.ie/press/releases/2012/20120224.html>.

Department of Health (2012e), 'Special Delivery Unit and National Treatment Purchase Fund', press release, 25 January 2012, <http://www.dohc.ie/press/releases/2012/20120125.html>.

Department of Health (2012f), *Interim Report of the Steering Group on the Review of the Mental Health Act 2001*, Dublin: Department of Health.

Department of Health (2012g), 'Legislation for New Directorate Structure in the HSE to Be in Place During the Summer', press release, 29 May 2012, <http://www.dohc.ie/press/releases/2012/20120529.html>.

Department of Health (2012h), 'Minister for Health Sets Out a New Policy Direction for Public Hospital Groups', press release, 30 March 2012, <http://www.dohc.ie/press/releases/2012/20120330.html>.

Department of Health (2012i), 'Reform Works – More on the Way', press release, 25 January 2012, <http://www.dohc.ie/press/releases/2012/20120125.html>.

Department of Health (2012j), 'Statement on Health Service Executive (Governance) Bill 2012', press release, 18 July 2012, <http://www.dohc.ie/press/releases/2012/20120718.html>.

Department of Health (2012k), 'Minister for Health Announces New Director General for HSE', 27 July 2012, <http://www.dohc.ie/press/releases/2012/20120727.html>.

Department of Health (2012l), *Department of Health Statement of Strategy 2011–2014*, Dublin: Department of Health.

Department of Health (2012m), 'Minister Reilly Announces Publication of the Department of Health Statement of Strategy 2011–2014', press release, 8 May 2012, <http://www.dohc.ie/press/releases/2012/20120508.html>.

Department of Health (2012n), 'Review of Undergraduate Nursing and Midwifery Degree Programmes', Consultation Report, 28 March 2012, Dublin: Department of Health.

Department of Health (2012o), 'National Cancer Control Programme Fact Sheet', Dublin: Department of Health, <http://www.dohc.ie/fact_sheets/>.

Department of Health (2012p), 'Minister Lynch Publishes Interim Report on the Review of the Mental Health Act 2001', press release, 21 June 2012, <http://www.dohc.ie/press/releases/2012/20120621.html>.

Department of Health (2012q), 'Minister Lynch Welcomes the Publication of the Mental Health Commission Annual Report for 2011', press release, 4 April 2012, <http://www.dohc.ie/press/releases/2012/20120404.html>.

Department of Health (2012r), *Value for Money and Policy Review of Disability Services in Ireland*, Dublin: Department of Health.

Department of Health (2012s), 'Free GP Care for Persons with Defined Long-term Illnesses', press release, 8 March 2012, <http://www.dohc.ie/press/releases/2012/20120308.html>.

Department of Health (2012t), *Future Health: A Strategic Framework for Reform of the Health Service 2012–2015*, Dublin: Department of Health.

Department of Health (UK) (2006), *NHS Foundation Trusts: A Source for Developing Governance Arrangements*, Version D: 12 January 2006, London: Department of Health.

Department of Health (UK) (2008), *High Quality Care: NHS Next Stage Review Final Report*, London: Her Majesty's Stationery Office.

Department of Health (UK) (2009), *Valuing People Now: A New Three-Year Strategy for People with Learning Disabilities*, London: Her Majesty's Stationery Office.

Department of Health (UK) (2010), *Essence of Care 2010: Benchmarks for the Fundamental Aspects of Care*, Norwich: Her Majesty's Stationery Office.

Department of Health (UK) (2010), *Midwifery 2020 Programme: Core Role of the Midwife Workstream Final Report*, London: Her Majesty's Stationery Office.

Department of Health and Children (1996), *A Management Development Strategy for the Health and Personal Social Services in Ireland*, Dublin: Department of Health and Children.

Department of Health and Children (1998), *Strategy Statement 1998–2001: Working for Health and Well-Being*, Dublin: Department of Health and Children.

Department of Health and Children (1999a), *SI No 376 of 1999 – National Council for the Professional Development of Nursing and Midwifery, Establishment Order, 1999*, Dublin: Stationery Office.

Department of Health and Children (1999b), *Children First: National Guidelines for the Protection and Welfare of Children*, Dublin: Stationery Office.

Department of Health and Children (2000a), *The National Children's Strategy: Our Children – Their Lives*, Dublin: Stationery Office.

Department of Health and Children (2000b), *Report of the Paediatric Nurse Education Group*, Dublin: Department of Health and Children, Nursing Policy Division.

Department of Health and Children (2001a), *Quality and Fairness: A Health System for You*, Dublin: Department of Health and Children.

Department of Health and Children (2001b), *Primary Care: A New Direction*, Dublin: Department of Health and Children.

Department of Health and Children (2001c), *Effective Utilisation of Professional Skills of Nurses and Midwives*, Dublin: Department of Health and Children.

Department of Health and Children (2002), *Action Plan for People Management*, Dublin: Department of Health and Children.

Department of Health and Children (2003a), *Report of the National Task Force on Medical Staffing* (The Hanly Report), Dublin: Department of Health and Children.

Department of Health and Children (2003b), *The Health Service Reform Programme*, Dublin: Department of Health and Children.

Department of Health and Children (2003c), *A Research Strategy for Nursing and Midwifery in Ireland: Final Report*, Dublin: Stationery Office.

Department of Health and Children (2003d), 'Report of the National Task Force on Medical Staffing 2003: The Challenge for Nursing and Midwifery', a discussion paper, Dublin: Department of Health and Children.

Department of Health and Children (2003e), *Nurses' and Midwives' Understanding and Experiences of Empowerment in Ireland*, Dublin: Department of Health and Children, Nursing Policy Division.

217

Department of Health and Children (2003f), *Evaluation of the Irish Pilot Programme for the Education of the Health Care Assistants*, Dublin: Department of Health and Children.

Department of Health and Children (2004a), *Health Information: A National Strategy*, Dublin: Department of Health and Children.

Department of Health and Children (2004b), *Report of the Expert Group on Midwifery and Children's Nursing Education*, Dublin: Stationery Office.

Department of Health and Children (2004c), *SI No 494 of 2004 – European Communities (Organisation of Working Time) (Activities of Doctors in Training) Regulations 2004*, Dublin: Stationery Office.

Department of Health and Children (2005a), *Policy Challenges: Obesity – Report of the National Taskforce on Obesity*, Dublin: Department of Health and Children.

Department of Health and Children (2005b), *Reach Out: National Strategy for Action on Suicide Prevention*, Dublin: Stationery Office.

Department of Health and Children (2006a), *A Vision for Change: Report of the Expert Group on Mental Health Policy*, Dublin: Stationery Office.

Department of Health and Children (2006b), *A Strategy for Cancer Control in Ireland*, Dublin: Department of Health and Children.

Department of Health and Children (2007a), *The Agenda for Children's Services: A Policy Handbook*, Dublin: Stationery Office.

Department of Health and Children (2007b), *SI No 201 of 2007 – Medicinal Products (Prescription and Control of Supply) (Amendment) Regulations 2007*, Dublin: Stationery Office.

Department of Health and Children (2008a), *Building a Culture of Patient Safety: The Report of the Commission on Patient Safety and Quality Assurance* (The Madden Report), Dublin: Stationery Office.

Department of Health and Children (2008b), *Tackling Chronic Disease: A Policy Framework for the Management of Chronic Disease*, Dublin: Department of Health and Children.

Department of Health and Children (2008c), *National Strategy for Service User Involvement in the Irish Health Service 2008–2013*, Dublin: Department of Health and Children.

Department of Health and Children (2009a), *Research Strategy for Nursing and Midwifery in Ireland 2003–2008: Review of Attainments*, Dublin: Department of Health and Children.

Department of Health and Children (2009b), *National Disability Strategy Towards 2016: Strategic Document*, <http://www.dohc.ie/publications/nds_strategy.html>.

Department of Health and Children (2009c), *Palliative Care for Children with Life-Limiting Conditions in Ireland: A National Policy*, Dublin: Stationery Office.

Department of Health and Children (2010a), 'Nurses and Midwives Bill: Regulatory Impact Analysis', <http://www.dohc.ie/otherhealth issues/nursesandmidwives/>.

Department of Health and Children (2010b), *State of the Nation's Children: Ireland 2010*, Dublin: Government Publications.

Department of Health and Children (2010c), *Changing Cardiovascular Health: National Cardiovascular Health Policy 2010–2019*, Dublin: Government Publications.

Department of Health and Children (2010d), *A Review of Practice Development in Nursing and Midwifery in the Republic of Ireland and the Development of a Strategic Framework*, Dublin: Department of Health and Children.

Department of Health and Children (2011a), *Strategic Framework for Role Expansion of Nurses and Midwives: Promoting Quality Patient Care*, Dublin: Stationery Office.

Department of Health and Children (2011b), 'Mental Health Services Fact Sheet', <htpp://www.dohc.ie/factsheets/mhsfactsheetjan2011.pdf?direct>.

Department of Health and Children (2011c), *Your Health Is Your Wealth: A Policy Framework for a Healthier Ireland 2012–2020*, Dublin: Department of Health and Children.

Department of Health and Health Service Executive (2012), *National Healthcare Charter: You and Your Health Service*, Dublin: Health Service Executive.

Department of Health and Children and Health Service Executive (2008), *Service User Involvement in the Irish Health Service: A Review of the Evidence*, Dublin: Department of Health and Children.

Department of Health and Children and Health Service Executive (2009), *An Integrated Workforce Planning Strategy for the Health Services 2009–2012*, Dublin: Health Service Executive.

Department of Justice and Law Reform (2004), 'National Disability Strategy', <http://www.justice.ie/en/JELR/NDS.pdf/files/NDS.pdf>.

Det Norske Veritas Ltd (2008), *Right Care, Right Place, Right Time: Advice on the Development of Paediatric Critical Care Facilities and Services in the Dublin Children's Hospitals between Now and the Completion of the National Paediatric Hospital*, London: Veritas Ltd.

Devane, D., Brennan, M., Begley, C., Clarke, M., Walsh, D., Sandall, J., Ryan, P., Revill, P. and Normand, C. (2010), *Socioeconomic Value of the Midwife: A Systematic Review, Meta-Analysis, Meta-Synthesis and Economic Analysis of Midwife-Led Models of Care*, London: Royal College of Midwives.

Domiciliary Birth Expert Group (2004), *Report to the Chief Executive Officers of the Health Boards*, Dublin: Health Service Executive.

Donald, F., Bryant-Lukosius, D., Martin-Misener, R., Kaasalainen, S., Kilpatrick, K., Carter, N., Harbman, P., Bourgeault, I. and DiCenso, A. (2010), 'Clinical Nurse Specialists and Nurse Practitioners: Title Confusion and Lack of Role Clarity', *Nursing Leadership* (Toronto, ON), December, 23 Spec No 2010:189-201.

Dooley, B. and Fitzgerald, A. (2012), *My World Survey: National Study of Youth Mental Health in Ireland*, Dublin: UCD School of Psychology; Dublin: Headstrong – The National Centre for Youth Mental Health.

Dublin Hospital Initiative Group (1991), *Reports (Three) of the Dublin Hospital Initiative Group 1990–1991*, Dublin: Stationery Office.

Dunham, J. and Klafehn, K. (1990), 'Transformational Leadership and the Nurse Executive', *Journal of Nursing Administration*, 20(4): 28–33.

Economic and Social Research Institute (ESRI) and Trinity College Dublin (2012), 'Growing Up in Ireland', <http://www.growingup.ie/>.

Elliott, N., Higgins, A., Begley, C., Lalor, J., Sheerin, F., Coyne, I. and Murphy, K. (2012), 'The Identification of Clinical and Professional Leadership Activities of Advanced Practitioners: Findings from the Specialist Clinical and Advanced Practitioner Evaluation Study in Ireland', *Journal of Advanced Nursing*, 00(0): 000–000, doi: 10.1111/j.1365-2648.2012.06090.x.

European Commission (2005a), *Directive 2005/36/EC of the European Parliament and of the Council of 7 September 2005 on the Recognition of Professional Qualifications*, Strasbourg: European Council and European Parliament.

European Commission (2005b), 'Improving the Mental Health of the Population: Towards a Strategy on Mental Health for the European Union' (Green Paper), Brussels: European Countries.

European Commission (2006), *Council Directive 2006/100/EC of 20 November 2006 Adopting Certain Directives in the Field of Freedom of Movement of Persons, by Reason of the Accession of Bulgaria and Romania*, Strasbourg: European Council and European Parliament.

European Commission (2011), 'Modernising the Professional Qualifications Directive (Directive 2005/36/EC)', Green Paper, Brussels: European Commission, <http://eur-lex.europa.eu/LexUriServ/LexUriServ.do?uri=COM:2011:0367:FIN:en:PDF>.

Expert Reference Group on Disability Policy (2011), *Report of Disability Policy Review*, <http://www.dohc.ie/publications/pdf/ERG_Disability_Policy_Review_Final.pdf?direct=I>.

Farrelly, M. (2008), *Concepts of Psychiatric/Mental Health Nursing in Psychiatric/Mental Health Nursing: An Irish Perspective*, Dublin: Gill & Macmillan.

References

Fealy, G.M., Carney, M., Drennan, J., Treacy, M., Burke, J., O'Connell, D., Howley, B., Clancy, A., McHugh, A., Patton, D. and Sheerin, F. (2009), 'Models of Initial Training and Pathways to Registration: A Selective Review of Policy in Professional Regulation', *Journal of Nursing Management*, 17: 730–738.

Felce, D., Baxter, H., Lowe, K., Dunstan, F., Houston, H., Jones, G., Felce, J. and Kerr, M. (2008), 'The Impact of Repeated Health Checks for Adults with Intellectual Disabilities', *Journal of Applied Research in Intellectual Disabilities*, 21: 85–596.

Fleming, V. and Holmes, A. (2005), *Basic Nursing and Midwifery Education in Europe: A Report to the World Health Organisation Regional Office for Europe*, Denmark: WHO Regional Office for Europe.

Flynn, M. (1998), *Management in the Health Services: The Role of the Nurse*, A Report Prepared for the Commission on Nursing, Dublin: Stationery Office.

Foley, A. (2012), *Estimates of Average Adult Alcohol Consumption 2001–2011 and International Comparison*, Dublin: The Alcohol Beverage Federation of Ireland.

George, J. (1996), *Nursing Theories: The Base for Professional Nursing Practice* (4th edition), Norwalk, CT: Appleton and Lang.

Giovino, G.A., Mirza, S.A., Samet, M.J., Gupta, P.C., Jarvis, M.J., Bhala, N., Peto, R., Zatonski, W., Hsia, J., Morton, J., Palipudi, K.M. and Asma, S. for the Global Adult Tobacco Survey (GATS) Collaborative Group (2012), 'Tobacco Use in 3 Billion Individuals from 16 Countries: An Analysis of Nationally Representative Cross-Sectional Household Surveys', *The Lancet*, 380(9842): 668–679.

Glen, S. and Leiba, T. (eds.) (2001), *Multi-Professional Learning for Nurses*, Basingstoke: Palgrave Macmillan.

Government of Ireland (1919), *The Nurses Registration Act 1919*, Dublin: Stationery Office.

Government of Ireland (1950), *Nurses Act 1950*, Dublin: Stationery Office.

Government of Ireland (1961a), *Nurses Act 1961*, Dublin: Stationery Office.

Government of Ireland (1961b), *Health (Corporate Bodies) Act 1961*, Dublin: Stationery Office.

Government of Ireland (1970), *Health Act 1970*, Dublin: Stationery Office.

Government of Ireland (1985), *Nurses Act 1985*, Dublin: Stationery Office.

Government of Ireland (1988), *Data Protection Act 1988*, Dublin: Stationery Office.

Government of Ireland (1997), *Commission on Nursing Interim Report*, Dublin: Stationery Office.

Government of Ireland (1998), *Report of the Commission on Nursing: A Blueprint for the Future*, Dublin: Stationery Office.

References

Government of Ireland (2000), *Nursing Education Forum: A Strategy for a Pre-Registration Nursing Education Degree Programme*, Dublin: Stationery Office.

Government of Ireland (2001), *Mental Health Act 2001*, Dublin: Stationery Office.

Government of Ireland (2003), *Data Protection (Amendment) Act 2003*, Dublin: Stationery Office.

Government of Ireland (2004a), *Health Act 2004*, Dublin: Stationery Office.

Government of Ireland (2004b), 'Regulating Better' (White Paper), Dublin: Stationery Office.

Government of Ireland (2005a), *Health and Social Care Professionals Act 2005*, Dublin: Stationery Office.

Government of Ireland (2005b), *Disability Act 2005*, Dublin: Stationery Office.

Government of Ireland (2007a), *Medical Practitioners Act 2007*, Dublin: Stationery Office.

Government of Ireland (2007b), *Health Act 2007*, Dublin: Stationery Office.

Government of Ireland (2007c), *Irish Medicines Board (Miscellaneous Provisions) Act 2006 (Commencement) Order 2007*, Dublin: Stationery Office.

Government of Ireland (2008), *SI No 164/2008 – Recognition of the Professional Qualifications of Nurses and Midwives (Directive 2005/36/EC) Regulations, 2008*, Dublin: Stationery Office.

Government of Ireland (2010), *SI No 3 of 2010 – Health (An Bord Altranais) (Additional Functions) Order 2010*, Dublin: Stationery Office.

Government of Ireland (2011a), *Nurses and Midwives Act 2011*, Dublin: Stationery Office.

Government of Ireland (2011b), *SI No 219/2011 – Health and Children (Alteration of Name of Department and Title of Minister) Order 2011*, Dublin: Stationery Office.

Government of Ireland (2011c), *SI No 715 of 2011 – Nurses and Midwives Act 2011 (Commencement Order) 2011*, Dublin: Stationery Office.

Government of Ireland (2012a), *Assisted Decision-Making (Capacity) Bill 2012*, Dublin: Stationery Office.

Government of Ireland (2012b), *Health Service Executive (Governance) Bill 2012*, Dublin: Stationery Office.

Government of Ireland (2012c), *SI No 275 of 2012 – Nurses and Midwives Act 2011 (Commencement Order) 2012*, Dublin: Stationery Office.

Griffiths, R. (1983), *NHS Management Inquiry* (The Griffiths Report), London: Department of Health and Social Security.

Griffin, M. and Melby, V. (2006), 'Developing an Advanced Nurse Practitioner Service in Emergency Care: Attitude of Nurses and Doctors', *Journal of Advanced Nursing*, 56(3): 292–301.

Hanafin, S., Houston, A.M. and Cowley, S. (2002), 'Vertical Equity in Service Provision: A Model for the Irish Public Health Nursing Service', *Journal of Advanced Nursing*, 39(1): 68–76.

Harding Clark, M. (2006), *The Lourdes Hospital Inquiry*, Dublin: Health Service Executive.

Hart, G. (1985), 'College-Based Education: Background and Bugs', *The Australian Nurses Journal*, 15(4), 46–48.

Harvey, B. (2007), *Evolution of Health Services and Health Policy in Ireland*, Dublin: Combat Poverty Agency.

Hatem, M., Sandall, J., Devane, D., Soltani, H. and Gates, S. (2008), 'Midwife-Led Versus Other Models of Care for Childbearing Women', *Cochrane Database Systematic Review*, 4: CD004667.

Healthcare Improvement Scotland (2011), *Draft Healthcare Quality Standard: Assuring Person-Centred, Safe and Effective Care: Clinical Governance and Risk Management*, Edinburgh: Healthcare Improvement Scotland.

Health Information and Quality Authority (HIQA) (2008), *Corporate Plan 2008–2010*, Dublin: HIQA.

Health Information and Quality Authority (HIQA) (2009), *National Quality Standards for Residential Care Settings for Older People in Ireland*, Dublin: HIQA.

Health Information and Quality Authority (HIQA) (2010a), *Draft National Standards for Safer Better Care: Consultation Document*, September 2010, Dublin: HIQA.

Health Information and Quality Authority (HIQA) (2010b), *Guidance on Developing Key Performance Indicators and Minimum Data Sets to Monitor Healthcare Quality*, Dublin: HIQA.

Health Information and Quality Authority (HIQA) (2011a), *National Quality Assurance Criteria for Clinical Guidelines*, Dublin: HIQA.

Health Information and Quality Authority (HIQA) (2011b), *Guidelines for Evaluating the Clinical Effectiveness of Health Technologies*, Dublin: HIQA.

Health Information and Quality Authority (HIQA) (2012a), *A Guide to the National Standards for Safer Better Healthcare*, Dublin: HIQA.

Health Information and Quality Authority (HIQA) (2012b), *National Standards for Safer Better Healthcare*, Dublin: HIQA.

Health Information and Quality Authority (HIQA) (2012c), *Report of the Investigation into the Quality, Safety and Governance of the Care Provided by the Adelaide and Meath Hospital, Dublin, Incorporating the National Children's Hospital (AMNCH) for Patients who Require Acute Admission*, Dublin: HIQA.

Health Information and Quality Authority (HIQA) (2012d), *Your Guide to the National Standards for the Protection and Welfare of Children – For Health Service Executive, Children and Family Services*, Dublin: HIQA.

Health Information and Quality Authority (HIQA) (2012e), *National Standards for the Protection and Welfare of Children – For Health Service Executive Children and Family Services*, Dublin: HIQA.

Health Research Board (HRB) (2012), *Alcohol: Public Knowledge, Attitudes and Behaviours Report*, Dublin: HRB.

Health Service Executive (HSE) (2005a), *National Service Plan 2006*, Dublin: HSE.

Health Service Executive (HSE) (2005b), *Reach Out: A National Strategy for Action on Suicide Prevention*, Dublin: HSE.

Health Service Executive (HSE) (2005c,) *Maternity Services in the Eastern Region: A Strategy for the Future, 2005–2011*, Dublin: HSE.

Health Service Executive (HSE) (2006), *Transformation Programme 2007–2010*, Dublin: HSE.

Health Service Executive (HSE) (2007), 'eLearning Guru', <http://elearning_hseland_ietohm/default.asp>.

Health Service Executive (HSE) (2008a), *Corporate Plan 2008–2011*, Dublin: HSE.

Health Service Executive (HSE) (2008b), *Clinical Directorates: The Way Forward, Briefing on Appointment of Clinical Directors throughout the Health Service*, August 2008, HMI, <http://tinyurl.com/d5wgzv>.

Health Service Executive (HSE) (2008c), *National Integration: Local Responsibility*, HSE, <http://tinyurl.com/kmscxo>.

Health Service Executive (HSE) (2008d), 'New Consultant Contract and Clinical Directorates Are a Major Step Forward', press release, 29 August 2008, <http://tinyurl.com/ofaz28>.

Health Service Executive (HSE) (2008e), *Proposed Terms and Conditions for a Contract of Employment for Consultants Employed in the Public Health Service*, Dublin: HSE.

Health Service Executive (HSE) (2009a), *Clinical Directorates: Principles and Framework*, Dublin: HSE.

Health Service Executive (HSE) (2009b), *Achieving Excellence in Clinical Governance: A Distributed Clinical Leadership Model for the HSE – Ensuring the Health and Personal Social Care System Is in Good Hands*, Dublin: HSE.

Health Service Executive (HSE) (2009c), *Towards Excellence in Clinical Governance: A Framework for Integrated Quality, Safety and Risk Management across HSE Service Providers*, Dublin: HSE.

Health Service Executive (HSE) (2009d), 'Integrated Services Programme: Stage 1 Working Paper – Quality and Clinical Care Directorate', Dublin: HSE.

Health Service Executive (HSE) (2009e), *Education, Training and Research: Principles and Recommendations*, Dublin: HSE.

Health Service Executive (HSE) (2009f) *Framework for the Corporate and Financial Governance of the Health Service Executive: Codes of Standards and Behaviour, Document 2.1*, Dublin: HSE.

Health Service Executive (HSE) (2010a), *Achieving Excellence in Clinical Governance: Towards a Culture of Accountability*, Dublin: HSE.

Health Service Executive (HSE) (2010b), *Achieving Excellence in Clinical Governance: Service User Involvement*, Dublin: HSE.

Health Service Executive (HSE) (2010c), 'National Leadership and Innovation and Centre for Nursing and Midwifery', <http://www.hse.ie/eng/about/who/onmsd/leadership/>.

Health Service Executive (HSE) (2011a), *National Service Plan 2011*, Dublin: HSE.

Health Service Executive (HSE) (2011b), *Time to Move on from Congregated Settings: A Strategy for Community Inclusion*, Dublin: HSE.

Health Service Executive (HSE) (2012a), 'National Clinical Programmes', <http://www.hse.ie/eng/about/Who/clinical/natclinprog/>.

Health Service Executive (HSE) (2012b), *National Service Plan 2012*, Dublin: HSE.

Health Service Executive (HSE) (2012c), 'Mother and Infant Scheme', <http://www.hse.ie/eng/services/Find_a_Service/maternity/combinedcare.html>.

Health Service Executive (HSE) (2012d), *A Vision for Psychiatric/Mental Health Nursing: A Shared Journey for Mental Health Care in Ireland*, Dublin: HSE.

Health Service Executive (HSE) (2012e), 'Clinical Governance Information Leaflet: We Are All Responsible and Together We Are Creating a Safer Healthcare System', <http://www.hse.ie/eng/about/Who/Quality_and_clinicalCare/Clinicalgovernance/qpsleaflet.pdf>.

Health Service Executive (HSE) (2012f), 'Clinical Governance Development: An Assurance Check for Health Service Providers. We Are All Responsible and How Are We Doing?', <http://www.hse.ie/eng/about/Who/Quality_and_clinicalCare/Clinicalgovernance/assurancecheck.pdf>.

Health Service Executive and Irish Hospice Foundation (2008), *Palliative Care for All – Integrating Palliative Care into Disease Management Frameworks*, Dublin: Health Service Executive and Irish Hospice Foundation.

Health Service Executive (HSE) and the Royal College of Physicians in Ireland (2012), 'National Care of the Elderly Clinical Care Programme Briefing Note May 2012', Dublin: HSE and RCPI.

Health Service Executive (HSE), Royal College of Physicians of Ireland, Royal College of Surgeons in Ireland, Irish Association of Directors of Nursing and Midwifery, and the Therapy Professions Committee (2010), *Report of the National Acute Medicine Programme*, Dublin: HSE.

Health Service Executive (HSE), Royal College of Physicians of Ireland, Royal College of Surgeons in Ireland, Irish Association of Directors of Nursing and Midwifery, and the Therapy Professions Committee

(2011), *National Clinical Programmes Local Implementation Guidance Pack, June 2011, Version 1*, Dublin: HSE.

Health Service Executive (HSE), Directorate of Clinical Strategy and Programmes Health Service Executive, Irish Committee on Emergency Medical Training, Irish Association for Emergency Medicine, Irish National Board of the College of Emergency Medicine, Royal College of Surgeons in Ireland, Office of the Director of Nursing and Midwifery HSE, and the Therapy Professions Committee (2012), *The National Emergency Medicine Programme: A Strategy to Improve Safety, Quality, Access and Value in Emergency Medicine in Ireland*, Dublin: HSE.

Health and Social Care Regulatory Forum (2009), *Framework for Public and Service User Involvement in Health and Social Care in Ireland*, Dublin: Health and Social Care Regulatory Forum.

Heath, H. (2007), *Three Years On – Caring in Partnership: Older People and Nursing Staff Working towards the Future*, London: Royal College of Nursing.

Heath, P. (2002), *National Review of Nursing Education*, Canberry, ACT: Commonwealth of Australia.

Henderson, V. (1961), *Basic Principles of Nursing Care*, London: International Council of Nurses.

Henderson, V. (1966), *The Nature of Nursing: A Definition and Its Implications, Practice, Research, and Education*, New York, NY: Macmillan Company.

Hennessy, D.A., Rowland, H. and Buckton, K. (1993), 'The Corporate Role of the Nursing Director', *Journal of Nursing Management*, 1: 161–169.

Hennessy, D.A. and Gilligan, J.H. (1994), 'Identifying and Developing Tomorrow's Trust Nursing Directors', *Journal of Nursing Management*, 2: 37–45.

Hickey, I. (2004), 'Can We Reduce the Burden of Depression? The Australian Experience with Beyond Blue: The National Depression Initiative', *Australasian Psychiatry*, 12: 38–46.

Higgins, A., Begley, C., Timmons, F., McGonagle, I. and Nevin, M. (2010), *Nurse and Midwife Competency Determination and Competency Development Planning Toolkit*, Dublin: National Council.

Higher Education Authority (2012), *Towards a Future Higher Education Landscape*, Dublin: Higher Education Authority.

Hollowell, J., Puddicombe, D., Rowe, R., Linsell, L., Hardy, P., Stewart, M., Redshaw, M., Newburn, M., McCourt, C., Sandall, J., Macfarlane, A., Silverton, L. and Brocklehurst, P. on behalf of the Birthplace in England Collaborative Group (2011), *The Birthplace National Prospective Cohort Study of Perinatal and Maternal Outcomes by Planned Place of Births*, London: NHS National Institute for Health Research.

Huston, C. (2008), 'Preparing Nurse Leaders for 2020', *Journal of Nursing Management*, 16: 905–911.

References

Institute of Medicine (2010) *The Future of Nursing: Leading Change, Advancing Health*, <http://www.iom.edu/Reports/2010/The-Future-of-Nursing-Leading-Change-Advancing-Health.aspx>.

Institute of Obstetricians and Gynaecologists (2006), *The Future of Maternity and Gynaecology Services in Ireland 2006–2016*, Dublin: The Institute of Obstetricians and Gynaecologists.

International Confederation of Midwives (ICM) (2011), 'Global Standards for Midwifery Education', <http://www.unfpa.org/sowmy/resources/docs/standards/en/R429_ICM_2011_Global_Standards_for_Midwifery_Regulation_2011_ENG.pdf>.

International Council of Nurses (2011) *Leadership for Change^tm*, <http://www.icn.ch/pillarsprograms/leadership-for-change/>.

Irish Times (2012a), 'Number of Suicides in Ireland Rose 7% Last Year, CSO Figures Reveal', *Irish Times*, 12 July 2012.

Irish Times (2012b), 'Average Alcohol Consumption Falling Says Report', *Irish Times*, 15 May 2012.

Irish Times (2012c), 'Findings on Fatalities of Children in Care a Disgrace', *Irish Times*, 21 June 2012.

Irish Times (2012d), 'Kinsale Pilot Project Hoping to Reform Dementia Services', *Irish Times*, 20 August 2012.

Irish Times (2012e), 'Plan for Reform in All Its Details', *Irish Times Healthplus*, 17 April 2012.

Irish Times (2012f), 'Self Harm Linked to Lack of Adult Support', *Irish Times*, 16 May 2012.

Kelleher, A. and Musgrave, E. (2000), 'Sick Children's Nursing', in J. Robins (ed.), *Nursing and Midwifery in Ireland in the Twentieth Century*, Dublin: An Bord Altranais.

Kelly, F. and Kelly, C. (2011), *HRB Statistics 13: Annual Report of the National Intellectual Disability Database Committee 2010*, Dublin: Health Research Board.

Kennedy, D. (1991), *Reports of the Dublin Hospitals Initiative Group 1990–1991*, Dublin: Stationery Office.

Kennedy, F., McDonnell, A., Gerrish, K., Howarth, A., Pollard, C. and Redman, J. (2012), 'Evaluation of the Impact of Nurse Consultant Roles in the United Kingdom: A Mixed Method Systematic Literature Review', *Journal of Advanced Nursing*, 68(4): 721–742.

Kessler, R.C., Berglund, P., Demler, O., Jin, R., Merikangas, K.R. and Walters, E.E. (2005), 'Lifetime Prevalence and Age-of-Onset Distributions of DSM-IV Disorders in the National Comorbidity Survey Replication', *Archives of General Psychiatry*, 62: 593–602.

Kim-Cohen, J., Caspi, A., Moffitt, T.E., Harrington, H.L., Milne, B.J. and Poulton, R. (2003), 'Prior Juvenile Diagnoses in Adults with Mental Disorder: Developmental Follow-Back of a Prospective-Longitudinal Cohort', *Archives of General Psychiatry*, 60: 709–717.

Kinder, P. (2001), *Report of the Maternity Services Review Group*, Kells: North Eastern Health Board.

King's College London (2007), 'Points of Entry and Specialization in Nurse Education: International Perspectives', *Policy+5*, <http://www.kcl.ac.uk/schools/nursing/nnru/policy2007/issue5.html>.

Kitson, A. (1999), 'The Essence of Nursing', *Nursing Standard*, 13(23): 42–46.

Klakovich, M. (1995), 'Development and Psychometric Evaluation of the Reciprocal Empowerment Scale', *Journal of Nursing Measurement*, 3(2): 127–143.

KPMG (2008), *Independent Review of Maternity and Gynaecology Services in the Greater Dublin Area Final Report (GDA)*, Dublin: KPMG.

Kuokkanen, L. and Leino-Kilpi, H. (2000), 'Power and Empowerment in Nursing: Three Theoretical Approaches', *Journal of Advanced Nursing*, 31(1): 235–241.

Kuokkanen, L. and Leino-Kilpi, H. (2001), 'The Qualities of an Empowered Nurse and the Factors Involved', *Journal of Nursing Management*, 9: 273–280.

Labour Court (1997), Recommendation No. LRC 15450, CD/97/48, Dublin.

Laing, R.D. (1971), *The Politics of the Family and Other Essays*, New York, NY: Pantheon.

Laschinger, H.K.S., Wong, C., McMahon, L. and Kaufmann, C. (1999), 'Leader Behaviour Impact on Staff Nurse Empowerment, Job Tension and Work Effectiveness', *Journal of Nursing Administration*, 29(5): 28–39.

Laschinger, H.K.S. (2001), 'Impact of Structural and Psychological Empowerment on Job Strain in Nursing Work Settings', *Journal of Nursing Administration*, 31(5): 260–272.

Laschinger, H.K.S., Finnegan, J., Shamian, J. and Casier, S. (2001), 'Organisational Trust and Empowerment in Restructured Healthcare Settings', *Journal of Nursing Administration*, 30(9): 413–425.

Leahy-Warren, P. (1998), *Community Nursing: An International Perspective – A Report Prepared for the Commission on Nursing*, Dublin: Stationery Office.

Leahy-Warren, P. and Tyrrell, M.P. (1998), *Joint Appointments in Nursing: A Report Prepared for the Commission on Nursing*, Dublin: Stationery Office.

Leathard, A. (ed.) (2003), *Interprofessional Collaboration: From Policy to Practice in Health and Social Care*, London: Routledge.

Lewis, A., Saunders, N. and Fenton, K. (2002), 'The Magic Matrix of Clinical Governance', *British Journal of Clinical Governance*, 7(3): 150–153.

Lokhoff, J., Wegewijs, B., Durkin, K., Wagenaar, R., Gonzalez, J., Isaacs, A.K., dalle Rose, L.F.D. and Gobbi, M. (2010), *A Tuning Guide to Formulating Degree Programme Profiles: Including Programme Competences and Programme Learning Outcomes*, Bilbao: Tuning Association Spain.

Longley, M., Shaw, C. and Dolan, G. (2007), *Nursing: Towards 2015 Alternative Scenarios for Healthcare, Nursing and Nurse Education in the UK in 2015*, Commissioned by the Nursing and Midwifery Council, <http://www.nmc-uk.org/Documents/ResearchPapers/Nursing%20 towards%202015%20full%20report%20.pdf>.

Maben, J. and Griffiths, P. (2008), *Nurses in Society: Starting the Debate*, National Nursing Research Unit, London: King's College London.

Machell, S., Gough, P. and Steward, K. (2009) *From Ward to Board: Identifying Good Practice in the Business of Caring*, London: King's Fund.

MacLellan, K. (2007), 'Expanding Practice: Developments in Nursing and Career Pathways', *Nursing Management*, 14(3): 28–34.

MacLellan, K. (2010), 'Advanced Practice: Nursing in Ireland', in E.M. Sullivan-Mark, D.O. McGivern, J.A. Fairman and S.A. Greenberg (eds.), *Nurse Practitioners* (5th edition), New York, NY: Springer Publishing.

Madden Report *see* Department of Health and Children (2008a).

McCarron, M., Swinburne, J., Burke, E., McGlinchey, E., Mulryan, N., Andrews, V., Foran, S. and McCallion, P. (2011), *Growing Older with an Intellectual Disability in Ireland 2011: First Results from the Intellectual Disability Supplement to the Irish Longitudinal Study on Ageing*, Dublin: School of Nursing and Midwifery, Trinity College Dublin.

McGorry, P. (2005), 'Every Me and Every You: Responding to the Hidden Challenge of Mental Illness in Australia', *Australian Psychology*, 13(1): 3–15.

McKenna, H.P., Keeney, S. and Bradley, M. (2004), 'Nurse Leadership within Primary Care: The Perceptions of Community Nurses, GPs, Policy Makers and Members of the Public', *Journal of Nursing Management*, 12: 169–76.

Medel-Anonuevo, C., Ohsako, T. and Mauch, V. (2001), *Revisiting Lifelong Learning in 21st Century*, UNESCO Institute for Education.

Mental Health Commission (2007), *Quality Framework for Mental Health Services in Ireland*, Dublin: MHC.

Mental Health Commission (2012), *Mental Health Commission Annual Report 2011, Including the Report of the Inspector of Mental Health Services*, Dublin: MHC.

Mernagh, E. (2010) *Taking Stock: Ten Years of the Bologna Process in Ireland*, Dublin: Higher Education Authority and National Qualifications Authority Ireland.

Mudiwa, L. (2011), 'Hospital Trusts on the Horizon', *Irish Medical Times*, 19(08): 2011.

National Council of New Zealand (2010), *Report of the Review of the Education Programme Standards for the Registered Nurse Scope of Practice*, Wellington: National Council of New Zealand.

National Council for the Professional Development of Nursing and Midwifery (2002), *Guidelines on the Development of Courses Preparing*

Nurses and Midwives as Clinical Nurse/Midwife Specialists and Advanced Nurse/Midwife Practitioners, Dublin: National Council.

National Council for the Professional Development of Nursing and Midwifery (2003a), *Agenda for the Future Professional Development of Nursing and Midwifery*, Dublin: National Council.

National Council for the Professional Development of Nursing and Midwifery (2003b), *Guidelines for Health Service Providers for the Selection of Nurses and Midwives Who Might Apply for Financial Support in Seeking Opportunities to Pursue Further Education*, Dublin: National Council.

National Council for the Professional Development of Nursing and Midwifery (2004a), *Report on the Continuing Professional Development of Staff Nurses and Staff Midwives*, Dublin: National Council.

National Council for the Professional Development of Nursing and Midwifery (2004b), *An Evaluation of the Effectiveness of the Role of the Clinical Nurse/Midwife Specialist*, Dublin: National Council.

National Council for the Professional Development of Nursing and Midwifery (2005a), *Agenda for the Future Professional Development of Public Health Nursing*, Dublin: National Council.

National Council for the Professional Development of Nursing and Midwifery (2005b), *Clinical Nurse Specialists and Advanced Nurse Practitioner Roles in Emergency Departments: Position Paper*, Dublin: National Council.

National Council for the Professional Development of Nursing and Midwifery (2005c), *Service Needs Analysis for Clinical Nurse/Midwife Specialists and Advanced Nurse/Midwife Practitioners*, Dublin: National Council.

National Council for the Professional Development of Nursing and Midwifery (2005d), *A Study to Identify Research Priorities for Nursing and Midwifery in Ireland*, Dublin: National Council.

National Council for the Professional Development of Nursing and Midwifery (2005e), *The Development of Joint Appointments: A Framework for Irish Nursing and Midwifery*, Dublin: National Council.

National Council for the Professional Development of Nursing and Midwifery (2005f), *A Preliminary Evaluation of the Role of the Advanced Nurse Practitioner*, Dublin: National Council.

National Council for the Professional Development of Nursing and Midwifery (2005g), *An Evaluation of the Extent and Nature of Nurse-Led/Midwife-Led Services in Ireland*, Dublin: National Council.

National Council for the Professional Development of Nursing and Midwifery (2006a), *Clinical Nurse Specialist and Advanced Nurse Practitioner Roles in Intellectual Disability Nursing: Position Paper 2*, Dublin: National Council.

National Council for the Professional Development of Nursing and Midwifery (2006b), *Report on the Baseline Survey of Research Activity in Irish Nursing and Midwifery*, Dublin: National Council.

National Council for the Professional Development of Nursing and Midwifery (2006c), *Improving the Patient Journey: Understanding Integrated Care Pathways*, Dublin: National Council.

National Council for the Professional Development of Nursing and Midwifery (2006d), *Measurement of Nursing and Midwifery Interventions: Guidance and Resource Pack*, Dublin: National Council.

National Council for the Professional Development of Nursing and Midwifery (2007a), *Clinical Nurse Specialist and Advanced Nurse Practitioner Roles in Older Persons Nursing: Position Paper 3*, Dublin: National Council.

National Council for the Professional Development of Nursing and Midwifery (2007b), *Criteria and Processes for the Allocation of Additional Funding for Continuing Education by the National Council* (2nd edition), Dublin: National Council.

National Council for the Professional Development of Nursing and Midwifery (2008a), *Framework for the Establishment of Clinical Nurse Specialist and Clinical Midwife Specialist Posts* (4th edition), Dublin: National Council.

National Council for the Professional Development of Nursing and Midwifery (2008b), *A Framework for the Establishment of Advanced Nurse Practitioner and Advanced Midwife Practitioner Posts* (4th edition), Dublin: National Council.

National Council for the Professional Development of Nursing and Midwifery (2008c), *Accreditation of Advanced Nurse Practitioners and Advanced Midwife Practitioners* (2nd edition), Dublin: National Council.

National Council for the Professional Development of Nursing and Midwifery (2008d), *Enhanced Nursing Practice in Emergency Departments: Position Paper 4*, Dublin: National Council.

National Council for the Professional Development of Nursing and Midwifery (2008e), *Enhanced Midwifery Practice: Position Paper 5*, Dublin: National Council.

National Council for the Professional Development of Nursing and Midwifery (2008f), *Role of the Nurse or Midwife in Medical-Led Research*, Dublin: National Council.

National Council for the Professional Development of Nursing and Midwifery (2008g), *Clinical Supervision – A Structured Approach to Best Practice: Discussion Paper 1*, Dublin: National Council.

National Council for the Professional Development of Nursing and Midwifery (2009a), *Guidelines for the Development of Portfolios for Nurses and Midwives* (3rd edition), Dublin: National Council.

National Council for the Professional Development of Nursing and Midwifery (2009b), *Service Needs Analysis: Informing Business and Service Plans*, Dublin: National Council.

National Council for the Professional Development of Nursing and Midwifery (2009c), *Guidance on the Adaptation of Clinical Practice Guidelines: Getting Evidence into Practice*, Dublin: National Council.

National Council for the Professional Development of Nursing and Midwifery (2009d), *Review of Achievements 1999–2009*, Dublin: National Council.

National Council for the Professional Development of Nursing and Midwifery (2010a), *Review of Achievements 1999–2010 – Publications: Leadership, Guidance and Evidence for Best Practice*, Dublin: National Council.

National Council for the Professional Development of Nursing and Midwifery (2010b), *Clinical Outcomes – Promoting Patient Safety and Quality of Care; Implications for Nurses and Midwives: Discussion Paper 2*, Dublin: National Council.

National Council for the Professional Development of Nursing and Midwifery (2010c), *Key Performance Indicators: A Guide to Choosing and Using KPIs for Clinical Nurse/Midwife Specialists and Advanced Nurse/Midwife Practitioners: Discussion Paper 3*, Dublin: National Council.

National Council for the Professional Development of Nursing and Midwifery (2010d), *Profiles of Advanced Nurse/Midwife Practitioners and Clinical Nurse//Midwife Specialists in Ireland* (2nd edition), Dublin: National Council.

National Council for the Professional Development of Nursing and Midwifery and the Health Service Executive South (2008), *Clinical Nurse/ Midwife Specialists Resource Pack* (2nd edition), Dublin and Kilkenny: National Council and HSE South.

National Health Service (2010), 'Health Needs Annual Evidence Update 2010', <http://www.library.nhs.uk/learningdisabilities/ViewResource.aspx?resID=317947>.

National Health Service Quality Improvement Scotland (2006), *Promoting Access to Healthcare for People with a Learning Disability: A Guide for Frontline NHS Staff*, Edinburgh: NHS Quality Improvement.

National Institute for Health and Clinical Excellence (NICE) (2007), 'About Clinical Guidelines', <http://www.nice.org.uk/guidance/index.jsp>.

National Paediatric Hospital Board (2010), 'National Model of Care for Paediatric Healthcare in Ireland', <http://www.newchildrenshospital.ie/index/ViewResource.aspx?resID=31794>.

National Paediatric Hospital Board (2012), 'Project Overview', <http://www.newchildrenshospital.ie/index.cfm/page/_project_overview>.

National Qualification Authority Ireland (2010), 'Tuning Educational Structures in Europe: A Pilot Project Supported by the European Commission in the Framework of the Socrates Programme', <http://www.nqai.ie>.

National Suicide Research Foundation (NSRF) (2012a), *National Registry of Deliverate Self Harm Ireland: Deliberate Self Harm in the Republic of Ireland – Annual Report 2011*, Cork: NSRF.

National Suicide Research Foundation (NSRF) (2012b), *First Report of the Suicide Support and Information System*, Cork: NSRF.

National Task Force on Suicide (1998), *Report of the National Task Force on Suicide*, Dublin: Stationery Office.

National Treatment Purchase Fund (NTPF) (2010), *Annual Report 2010*, Dublin: NTPF.

Nelson, S. and Gordon, S. (2005), *The Complexities of Care: Nursing Reconsidered*, New York, NY: Cornell University Press.

Neuman, B. (1995), *The Neuman Systems Model* (3rd edition), Norwalk, CT: Appleton & Lang.

Nightingale, F. (1860), *Notes on Nursing: What It Is and What It Is Not*, New York, NY: D. Appleton & Company.

North Eastern Health Board (NEHB) (2001), *Report of the Maternity Services Review Group*, Drogheda: North Eastern Health Board.

Nursing and Midwifery Council (NMC) (2004), *Pre-Registration Midwifery Education Review Report*, London: NMC.

Nursing and Midwifery Council (NMC) (2009), *Standards for Pre-Registration Midwifery Education*, London: NMC.

Nursing and Midwifery Council (NMC) (2010), *Standards for Pre-Registration Nursing Education*, London: NMC.

O'Connell, F. (2008), 'Sharing the Care of COPD', *Irish Medical Times*, 40.

Office for Health Management (OHM) (2000), 'Report on Nursing Management Competencies', <http://www.pndhseland.ie/corp/ohmpublications/2000.html>.

Office for Health Management (OHM) (2001a), 'Clinicians in Management Discussion Paper 1: Introduction and Case Studies', <https://www.pnd.hseland.ie/corp/ohmpublications/2001.html>.

Office for Health Management (OHM) (2001b), 'Clinicians in Management Discussion Paper 2: A Framework for Discussion', <https://www.pnd.hseland.ie/corp/ohmpublications/2001.html>.

Office for Health Management (OHM) (2002a), 'Clinicians in Management Discussion Paper 3: A Review of the Initiative and Pointers to the Way Forward', <https://www.pnd.hseland.ie/corp/ohmpublications/2002.html>.

Office for Health Management (OHM) (2002b), 'Clinicians in Management Discussion Paper 4: A Review of Clinical Leadership', <https://www.pnd.hseland.ie/corp/ohmpublications/2002.html>.

Office for Health Management (OHM) (2003), 'Clinicians in Management Discussion Paper 5: Clinicians in Management at Work in Mayo General Hospital', <https://www.pnd.hseland.ie/corp/ohmpublications/2001.html>.

Office for Health Management (OHM) (2004), 'The Management Competency User Pack for Nurse and Midwife Managers', <https://www.pnd.hseland.ie/corp/ohmpublications/20041208002019.html>.

Office for Public Management (2001), *The Joint Appointments Guide: A Guide to Setting Up, Managing and Maintaining Joint Appointments for Health Improvements between Health Organisations and Local Government*, OPM.

Orem, D.E. (1985), *Nursing: Concepts of Practice* (3rd edition), New York, NY: McGraw Hill.

Organisation for Economic Co-operation and Development (OECD) (2010), 'Nurses in Advanced Roles: A Description and Evaluation of Experiences in 12 Developed Countries', Health Working Paper 54, Paris: OECD, <http://www.sourceoecd.org/els/health/working papers>.

O'Shea, E., Murphy, K., Larkin, P., Payne, S., Froggatt, K., Casey, D., Ni Leime, A. and Keys, M. (2008), *End-of-Life Care for Older People in Acute and Long-Stay Care Settings in Ireland*, Dublin: Hospice Friendly Hospitals Programme and National Council on Ageing and Older People.

O'Shea, E. and Kennelly, B. (2008), *The Economics of Mental Health Care in Ireland*, Dublin: Mental Health Commission.

O'Shea, Y. (1992), 'Quality Assurance in Nursing in a General Hospital: The Experience of St James's Hospital, Dublin', BA (Health Admin.) dissertation, Institute of Public Administration (IPA)/National Council for Educational Awards (NCEA) (unpublished).

O'Shea, Y. (1995), 'Resource Management and the Clinical Directorate Model: Implications for St James's Hospital Dublin', MSc Econ. dissertation, Trinity College Dublin (unpublished).

O'Shea, Y. (2008a), *Nursing and Midwifery in Ireland: A Strategy for Professional Development in a Changing Health Service*, Dublin: Blackhall Publishing.

O'Shea, Y. (2008b), 'Strengthening the Contribution of Nursing and Midwifery to Health and Healthcare in Ireland: A Strategy for Professional Development in a Changing Health Service', PhD thesis, Trinity College Dublin (unpublished).

O'Shea, Y. (2009), *Clinical Directorates in the Irish Health Services: Managing Resources and Patient Safety*, Dublin: Blackhall Publishing.

Our Lady's Hospital for Sick Children (2010), *Paediatric Intensive Care Unit 1st Annual Report (PICANet) 2010*, Dublin: Our Lady's Hospital for Sick Children.

Packwood, M., Keen, J. and Buxton, M. (1991), *Hospitals in Transition: The Resource Management Experiment*, Milton Keynes: Open University Press.

Prospectus Strategy Consultants (2003), *Audit of Structures and Functions in the Health System 2003* (The Prospectus Report), Dublin: Stationery Office.

Public Services Organisation Review Group (1969), *Report of the Public Services Organisation Review Group, 1966–1969* (The Devlin Report), Dublin: Stationery Office.

Pulcini, J., Jelic, M., Gul, R. and Loke, A.Y. (2010), 'An International Survey on Advanced Practice Nursing Education, Practice and Regulation', *Journal of Nursing Scholarship*, 42(1): 31–39.

Raferty, A.M., Clarke, S.P., Coles, J., Ball, J., James, P., McKee, M. and Aiken, L.H. (2007), 'Outcomes of Variation in Hospital Nurse Staffing in English Hospitals: Cross-Sectional Analysis of Survey Data and Discharge Records', *International Journal of Nursing Studies*, 44(2): 175–182.

Raines, C.F. and Taglaireni, E. (2008), 'Career Pathways in Nursing: Entry Points and Academic Progression', *Online Journal of Issues in Nursing*, 13(3).

Richardson, L. (1994), 'Writing: A Method of Inquiry', in N.K. Denzin and Y.S. Lincoln (eds.), *Handbook of Qualitative Research*, Thousand Oaks, CA: Sage.

RN4CAST Nurse Forecasting in Europe (2012a), 'Nurse Survey for Ireland Summary', Research Update No. 1 of 3. This research update was prepared by Ms Marcia Kirwan on behalf of the DCU RN4CAST Research Team: Professor A. Scott, Dr A. Mathews, Ms Marcia Kirwan, Ms Daniela Lehwaldt, Dr Roisin Morris and Professor Anthony Staines.

RN4CAST Nurse Forecasting in Europe (2012b), 'Patient Satisfaction with Nursing and Hospital Care in Irish General Hospitals', Research Update No. 2 of 3. This research update was prepared by Ms Marcia Kirwan on behalf of the DCU RN4CAST Research Team: Professor A. Scott, Dr A. Mathews, Ms Marcia Kirwan, Ms Daniela Lehwaldt, Dr Roisin Morris and Professor Anthony Staines.

RN4CAST Nurse Forecasting in Europe (2012c), 'Nurse Workforce Planning for the Nursing Profession: Current Perspectives and Recent Research Findings for Ireland', Research Update No. 3 of 3. This research update was prepared by Ms Marcia Kirwan on behalf of the DCU RN4CAST Research Team: Professor A. Scott, Dr A. Mathews, Ms Marcia Kirwan, Ms Daniela Lehwaldt, Dr Roisin Morris and Professor Anthony Staines.

Robinson, S. and Griffiths, P. (2007), *Nursing Education and Regulation: International Profiles and Perspectives*, London: King's College.

Rogers, C. (1976), *Introduction to Nursing: An Adaptation Model*, New York, NY: Prentice-Hall.

Roper, N., Logan, W.W. and Tierney, A.J. (2000), *The Roper-Logan-Tierney Model of Nursing: Based on Activities of Living*, Edinburgh: Elsevier Health Sciences.

Royal College of Nursing (1990), *Clinical Directorates and Nursing*, London: Royal College of Nursing.

Royal College of Nursing (2005), *RCN Manifesto: Nurses at Decision-Making Level*, London: Royal College of Nursing.

Royal College of Nursing (2006), *Meeting the Health Needs of People with Learning Disabilities: Guidance for Nursing Staff*, London: Royal College of Nursing.

Royal College of Nursing (2009), *RCN Policy Position: Executive Director of Nursing*, London: Royal College of Nursing.

Royal College of Nursing (2012), *Safe Staffing for Older People's Wards: RCN Summary Guidance and Recommendations*, London: Royal College of Nursing.

Royal College of Nursing and the British Geriatrics Society (2001), *Older People Specialist Nurse: A Joint Statement from the Royal College of Nursing and the British Geriatrics Society*, London: Royal College of Nursing and British Geriatrics Society.

Royal College of Physicians of Ireland National Immunisation Advisory Committee (2008), *Immunisation Guidelines for Ireland* (online September 2011), Dublin: Royal College of Physicians of Ireland.

St James's Hospital, Dublin (1996), 'Tender for the Establishment and Provision of Cardiac Surgery Services at St James's Hospital'.

Savage, E.B. (1998), *An Examination of the Changes in the Professional Role of the Nurse Outside Ireland, 1980–1997: A Report Prepared for the Commission on Nursing*, Dublin: Stationery Office.

Scoble, K. and Russell, G. (2003), 'Vision 2020, Part 1: Profile of the Future Nurse Leader', *Journal of Nursing Administration*, 33(6): 324–330.

Scott, P.A., Hayes, E. and MacNeela, P. (2006), *An Exploration of the Core Nursing Elements of Care Provided by Registered General Nurses Within the Community Setting*, Dublin: Dublin City University.

Sermeus, W., Aiken, L.H., Van den Heede, K., Rafferty, A.M., Griffiths, P., Moreno-Casbas, M.T., Busse, R., Lindqvist, R., Scott, A.P., Bruyneel, L., Brzostek, T., Kinnunen, J., Schubert, M., Schoonhoven, L., Zikos, D. and RN4CAST Consortium (2011), 'Nurse Forecasting in Europe (RN4CAST): Rationale, Design and Methodology', *BMC Nursing*, 10: 6, <http://www.biomedcentral.com/1472-6955/10/6>.

Severs, M. and Bowers, H. (1993), 'Management of Nursing Services within Clinical Directorates', in A. Hopkins (ed.), *The Role of Hospital Consultants in Clinical Directorates*, London: Royal College of Physicians.

Sheer, B. and Wong, F.K.Y. (2008), 'The Development of Advanced Nursing Practice Globally', *Journal of Nursing Scholarship*, 40(3): 204–211.

Sheridan, A. (2000), 'Psychiatric Nursing', in J. Robins (ed.), *Nursing and Midwifery in Ireland in the Twentieth Century*, Dublin: An Bord Altranais.

Simons, H., Clarke, J.B., Gobbi, M., Long, G., Mountford, M. and Wheelhouse, C. (1998), *Nurse Education and Training Evaluation in Ireland: Independent External Evaluation (Final Report)*, Southampton: University of Southampton.

Sofarelli, D. (1998), 'The Need for Nursing Leadership in Uncertain Times', *Journal of Nursing Management*, 6(4): 201–207.

Sullivan-Mark, E.M., McGivern, D.O., Fairman, J.A. and Greenberg, S.A. (eds.) (2010), *Nurse Practitioners* (5th edition), New York, NY: Springer Publishing.

Titchen, A. (1998), 'Professional Craft Knowledge in Patient-Centred Nursing and the Facilitation of Its Development', DPhil thesis, Department of Education Studies, University of Oxford (unpublished).

Tyrrell, M.P. (1998), *Developments in Pre-Registration Nursing Education: An International Perspective*, A Report Prepared for the Commission on Nursing, Dublin: Stationery Office.

United Nations (2006), *Final Report of the Ad Hoc Committee on a Comprehensive and Integral International Convention on the Protection and Promotion of the Rights and Dignity of Persons with Disabilities*, New York, NY: United Nations.

United Nations (2008), *Convention on the Rights of Persons with Disabilities*, New York, NY: United Nations.

Upenieks, V. (2003), 'Nurse Leaders' Perceptions of What Comprises Successful Leadership in Today's Acute Inpatient Environment', *Nursing Administration Quarterly*, 27(2): 140–152.

Van Schrojenstein Lantman-de Valk, H. and Noonan Walsh, P. (2008), 'Managing Health Problems in People with Intellectual Disabilities', *British Medical Journal*, 1408–1412.

Victoria Government Department of Human Sciences (2005), *Better Quality, Better Health Care*, Melbourne, VA: Victoria Government Department of Human Sciences.

Walker, D. (1993), 'Benefits of Clinical Directorates', in A. Hopkins (ed.), *The Role of Hospital Consultants in Clinical Directorates*, London: Royal College of Physicians.

West, E. and Rafferty, A.M. (2004), *The Future Nurse: Evidence of the Impact of Registered Nurses*, York: University of York.

Wood, V. (2008), *Nurses in Society: Starting the Debate, Oral Evidence*, London: Lala & Wood.

Working Group on the Effective Utilisation of Professional Skills of Nurses and Midwives (2001), *Report of the Working Group on the*

Effective Utilisation of Professional Skills of Nurses and Midwives, Dublin: Department of Health and Children.

Working Party on General Nursing (1980), *Report of the Working Party on General Nursing*, Dublin: Stationery Office.

World Health Organisation (WHO) (1981), *Global Strategy for Health for All by the Year 2000*, Geneva: WHO.

World Health Organisation (WHO) (1996), *Nursing Practice: Report of a WHO Expert Committee*, Geneva: WHO.

World Health Organisation (WHO) (2001a), *Nurses and Midwives for Health: WHO European Strategy for Nursing and Midwifery Education*, Copenhagen: WHO Regional Office.

World Health Organisation (WHO) (2001b), *The World Health Report 2001: Mental Health: New Understanding, New Hope*, Geneva: WHO.

World Health Organisation (WHO) (2003a), *What Are the Arguments for Community-Based Mental Health Care? HEN Report*, Geneva: WHO.

World Health Organisation (WHO) (2003b), *Investing in Mental Health*, Geneva: WHO.

World Health Organisation (WHO) (2004a), *The Solid Facts – Palliative Care*, Copenhagen: WHO.

World Health Organisation (WHO) (2004b), *Better Palliative Care for Older People*, Copenhagen: WHO.

World Health Organisation (WHO) (2004c), *World Health Report 2004*, Geneva: WHO.

World Health Organisation (WHO) (2005), 'Suicide Prevention', <http://www.who.int/mentalhealth/prevention/suicide/suicideprevent/en/index.html>.

World Health Organisation (WHO) (2006), *Dollars, DALYs and Decisions: Economic Aspects of the Mental Health System*, Geneva: WHO.

World Health Organisation (WHO) (2009), *Global Standards for the Initial Education of Professional Nurses and Midwives*, Geneva: WHO.

World Health Organisation (WHO, on behalf of the European Observatory on Health Systems and Policies) (2010), *Tackling Chronic Disease in Europe: Strategies, Interventions and Challenges*, Copenhagen: WHO Regional Office for Europe.

World Health Organisation (WHO) (2011), *Palliative Care for Older People: Better Practices*, Copenhagen: WHO.

INDEX

Note: The letter 'f' following a page number indicates a figure and 't' indicates a table.

Index